Internal Diseases of Domestic Animals

INTERNAL DISEASES OF DOMESTIC ANIMALS

Dr. Bernard Malkmus

2025

BIOTECH BOOKS

First Indian Edition 2025

ISBN 978-81-7622-076-7

Published by : **BIOTECH BOOKS**
4762-63/23, Ansari Road, Darya Ganj,
New Delhi - 110002
Phones : 011 4300 3222
Email : biotechbooks@yahoo.co.in

PRINTED IN INDIA

Authorized Translation

Translator's Preface.

IN the translation of Malkmus' "Grundriss der Klinischen Diagnostik" we have endeavored simply to reproduce the author's ideas with the hope that the English and American Veterinary Students may thus be provided with a text-book for which they have long felt a need. The needs of the students in the College of Veterinary Medicine of the Ohio State University have been the direct cause of the hurried undertaking of this work. A few short notes which we thought proper to add here and there, throughout the book, have been placed in [ ].

DAVID S. WHITE,
PAUL FISCHER.

Author's Preface to the Fourth Edition.

The present fourth edition has undergone in all departments a thorough revision. A few new cuts have been added, some of which graphically demonstrate the respirations by instructive curves. Throughout I have endeavored not only to furnish the student an adequate guide but also to provide the practitioner with a reliable adviser.

Notwithstanding the numerous additions, by increasing the amount of printed matter on each page, the former handy size of the book has been retained. MALKMUS.

Preface to First Edition

THE only safe foundation for the treatment of animal diseases is a correct diagnosis of the malady. In therapeutic as well as in forensic veterinary medicine everything depends on a correct recognition of the disease. This is the most difficult part of veterinary medicine, and methodical training alone will enable the student to develop into a practicing veterinarian who can do justice to this demand.

The following little work which offers a great variety of material in a most condensed form is intended as a guide for the diagnostician in recognizing and understanding the symptoms of disease. Although it represents the result not only of personal, but of veterinary experience in general, for the sake of clearness and general appearance the names of the numerous authors have been omitted. The results of bacteriological research which have an important bearing on diagnostics have been given due prominence. I have also deemed it appropriate to call attention, at the proper places, to those diseases or conditions which are considered as factors in annulling, or setting aside a sale. It was necessary to append a brief description of the most common diseases in order to give the student a general idea of the character of the maladies that affect the various functional apparatus, thus refreshing his memory and enabling him to institute comparisons between what he learns from his lectures and sees in the clinic.

The true to life representations of the horse and cow, which are copied from the "Handbuch der Anatomie der Thiere für Künstler," I owe to the kindness of Prof. Dr. Ellenberger and Prof. Dr. Baum of Dresden. I here most kindly thank these gentlemen for their unselfish obligingness.

The publishing house of Gebrüder Jänecke have disregarded both expense and trouble in order to supply good illustrations and to give the book a neat appearance; to them, too, my gratitude is due.

Hanover, November, 1898. MALKMUS.

Table of Contents.

	PAGE
The Diagnosis of Diseases	11
Symptoms	12
Determining the Diseased Organ	14
The Recognition of the Disease	15
I. Anamnesis	18
II. Determining the Status Praesens	21
Method of Examination.	
Inspection	21
Palpation	23
Percussion	24
Auscultation	29
A. General Part of Examination	31
1. Signalment	31
2. Habitus	32
I. Attitude of the Patient	33
II. Condition	39
III. Conformation	40
IV. Temperament	40
Diseases which are characterized particularly by change in Habitus	42
3. The Skin	3
I. Condition of the Hair Coat	44
II. The Skin's Moisture	45
III. Swellings in, and immediately under, the Skin	46
IV. Color of the Skin	49
V. Condition of the Skin	50
Diseases of the Skin	50

4. Examination of the Conjunctiva 59
I. Discharge from the Eyelids 60
II. Color 61
III. Swelling 63

5. Bodily Temperature 63
I. The Normal Temperature 65
II. Temperature of the Skin 66
III. Fever 66
IV. Subnormal Temperature 71
General Infectious Diseases 71

B. Special Part of the Examination. 75

6. Circulatory Apparatus 75
I. Pulse 75
II. Examination of the Peripheral Blood Vessels 81
III. The Heart 83
Diseases of the Circulatory Apparatus 91

7. Respiratory Apparatus 93
I. The Respiratory Movements 94
II. The Breath 105
III. Nasal Discharge 107
IV. The Nasal Cavities and Adjacent Sinuses 112
V. Examination of the Submaxillary Lymph Glands 115
VI. Cough 117
VII. The Voice 121
VIII. The Larynx and Trachea 122
IX. Percussion of the Thorax 124
X. Auscultation of the Lungs 130
Diseases of the Respiratory Apparatus 135

8. Digestive Apparatus 140
I. Food and Drink 140
II. The Buccal Cavity 146
III. The Throat and Esophagus 149

IV. Rumination 150
V. Vomiting 151
VI. The Abdomen 153
VII. Intestinal Discharges or Evacuations. 163
Diseases of Digestive Apparatus 171

9. Urinary Apparatus 176
I. Manner of Voiding the Urine....... 177
II. Examination of the Urine.......... 179
A. Macroscopical Examination..... 179
B. Chemical Examination.......... 182
C. Microscopical Examination...... 193
A. Crystalline Constituents of Urine 194
B. Organized Elements of Urine... 196
III. Examination of the Urinary Organs.. 199
Diseases of the Urinary Apparatus 201
Diseases of Tissue Metabolism.............. 202

10. The Sexual Apparatus 202
I. Abnormally Increased Sexual Appetite 202
II. The Vulva 203
III. The Vaginal Mucous Membrane..... 204
IV. The Udder 204
V. Diseases of the Male Sexual Organs. 206
Diseases of the Sexual Organs.. 207

11. The Nervous System........................ 208
I. Psychic Functions 210
II. Sensibility 212
III. Motility 213
Diseases of the Nervous System. 218

C. Specific Examinations. 221

12. Body Movements 221
I. Examination for Immobility......... 221
II. Examination for Heaves........... 224
III. Examination for Roaring........... 226
IV. Examination for Epilepsy and Vertigo 228
V. Examination for Balkiness......... 229

13. Diagnostic Inoculation 230

I. Tuberculosis 231
II. Glanders 235
III. Anthrax, Blackleg, Malignant Edema and Wild-und Rinder-Seuche 240
IV. Rabies 241

14. The Lymphatic Glands 243

15. The Blood 245

Diseases of the Blood 249

The Diagnosis of Diseases.

The object of practical veterinary medicine is manifold, but in the main it consists in the restoration of the destroyed health of our domestic animals. For this purpose a knowledge of the affected organ and of the character of the disease is indispensable, because this knowledge offers the only safe basis for a rational treatment and a correct prognosis.

Thus the art of making a correct diagnosis is not only the foundation upon which practical veterinary medicine rests, but it is pre-eminently that which elevates medicine to the dignity of a science.

Diagnosis is the art of determining internal changes of the body by the aid of externally visible or otherwise appreciable changes in the animal's condition or some of its organs. It also includes the recognition and name of the disease.

Since disease is a deviation from normal conditions and physiological processes, morbid changes cannot be recognized without a knowledge of normal conditions.

In the classroom the student has no opportunity to study the physical characteristics and the physiological functions of organs in living animals; he must learn this from personal observation and investigation in the clinic. In the clinic he must cultivate his senses and learn to hear, see, feel and smell in order to be able to judge correctly.

In the course of his practice different species of animals are presented to the veterinarian for clinical examination. This gives rise to certain difficulties which, in the main, are based on differences in anatomical structure and physiological function of the organs of different animals. The methods of examination are about the same for all species. One who has thoroughly learned the fundamental principles underlying the methods for the proper examination of a horse will have little trouble in adapting them to other animals. However, important differences in this respect will receive due consideration.

A further considerable difficulty in diagnostics, for the veterinarian, is his inability to determine the subjective feeling of a patient. Still, this is of less importance than the layman usually supposes. On the other hand, to compensate for this, we are in a position, in all cases, to make a complete objective examination of the patient in any direction. In this respect we have an advantage over the physician who is frequently denied this privilege and is, besides, liable to be misled by the imagination, whim, shame or vanity of the patient.

A diagnosis consists in the determination of

1. The symptoms of the disease.
2. The diseased organ.
3. The character of the disease—its name.

A Symptom is any observable deviation from the normal state or condition. Anatomy and physiology treat of the normal conditions and functions; *Symptomatology* treats of morbid conditions and of perverted functions.

The particular object of a clinical examination is the *determination of symptoms;* it must therefore include the external appearance and general behavior of the animal as well as a careful inspection of every accessible organ. To avoid mistakes or overlooking important factors we must conduct this examination according to a definite plan.

The best plan to follow is to take up the different functional apparatus in their physiological order and complete the examination of each in its turn. The beginner should memorize the scheme and follow it faithfully. This is no difficult task since the arrangement is a physiological and therefore natural one.

We propose the following order of procedure:

I. *Anamnesis* (ascertaining previous history of case).

II. *Determining the Status Praesens.*

A. General examination.

1. Signalment of the patient.
2. Habitus.
3. Skin.
4. Conjunctiva.
5. Temperature.

B. Special examinations.

6. Circulatory apparatus.
7. Respiratory apparatus.
8. Digestive apparatus.
9. Urinary apparatus.
10. Sexual apparatus.
11. Central nervous system.

C. Specific examinations.

12. Locomotion, exercise in harness or under saddle, etc.
13. Diagnostic inoculations.
14. Examination of lymphatic glands.
15. Examination of the blood.

The anamnesis should be procured and the general and special examination should be made at least once during the first visit to the patient. If the diseased organ or organs have been ascertained they must be carefully re-examined at every subsequent visit, at the same time we must be on the alert for the appearance of possible symptoms in other organs.

The specific examinations are made only when necessary for clinching the diagnosis.

The determination of symptoms is at times difficult.

Sometimes external influences bring about certain conditions of the healthy body which must not be interpreted as symptoms of disease, although they might, under other circumstances, be such; e. g., a horse refuses its feed—this is a frequent occurrence in gastro-intestinal affections or in the course of severe general diseases, but it may also be due to an excitable temperament of the animal or to the fact that the food in itself is undesirable—spoiled, mouldy. Hence the practitioner must always endeavor to determine the cause of the symptoms, whether the deviations from the normal are really due to disease or to external conditions.

The importance of symptoms depends very largely upon the conditions under which they appear.

Rapid respiratory movements may be due to a disease of the respiratory apparatus or to some other affection; again, they invariably occur after bodily exertions, and high temperatures, even when the animal is at perfect rest, will cause the respiratory movements to become accelerated.

To avoid confusing symptoms produced by muscular exercise, or other efforts on the part of the animal, with symptoms of disease, the patient should first be examined in a state of rest. Furthermore, all conditions that could possibly influence normal physiological processes must ever be taken into consideration; for example, we will mention age, estral period, pregnancy, fright on part of the animal, etc.

After noting the symptoms of the disease we come to the most difficult part of clinical diagnostics, viz:

The determination of the organ diseased. There are only a few symptoms which point with certainty to an affection of a definite organ, fewer still enable us to recognize the character of the disease; these latter are called *pathognomonic symptoms.* As a rule all symptoms must be first noted and then considered as a whole, always bearing in mind the principles of general and special pathology.

The symptoms which appear in a disease have for the determination of the affected organ a varied importance. *Local Symptoms* emanate from the diseased organ and therefore are noted only when certain organs are suffering. For this reason local symptoms are of great importance in diagnosis. *General symptoms* originate from the sympathy of the whole organism induced when varied organs are diseased. General symptoms may arise from the primary disease and be called (a) *direct* symptoms, or they may be due to complications or sequela when they are spoken of as (b) *indirect* or *accidental* symptoms.

To determine the affected organ all symptoms are carefully reconsidered in the order in which they were determined. The healthy apparatus are for the time being disregarded, the diseased apparatus are given special consideration.

A variation in the normal functional activity of an organ does not *in itself* indicate disease, it may simply be a compensatory variation (one due to an opposite variation in a similar organ) due to the primary morbid condition. The therapeutist's object is to ascertain the primarily affected organ, bring about a cure in this and secondarily cause the sympathetically affected organ to regain its natural condition and activity.

To discover the primarily affected organ requires a knowledge of the morbid processes that take place in each organ and of the local and general symptoms produced by them. This requirement is still more important for the final aim or ultimate purpose of diagnostics, viz:

The recognition of the disease itself according to kind, etiology, intensity and duration. The method of examination of each organ will therefore be followed by a short description of the most important diseases of each.

One who has not yet learned from his school training or practical experience, to appreciate the various symptoms which characterize each of the diseases and who has not a well-defined mental picture of the appearance of each of the diseases with which he must come in contact, will never become a good diagnostician.

Diagnosis *per se* has a different value depending upon whether it is made for a scientific or wholly practical purpose. It is often symptomatic and thus merely cloaks our ignorance; diabetes insipidus, colic, for instance. The purpose of diagnosis is more nearly attained when it includes the cause of the disease ("etiological diagnosis"), which is of value even if we do not know more of the cause than that it is some specific infection (influenza). An anatomical diagnosis is not conclusive because it does not indicate the cause (nasal catarrh, bowel catarrh). An ideal diagnosis would be "etiologico-anatomical" (skin glanders, acarus mange, verminous bronchitis). A correct prognosis and rational treatment are largely dependent upon a knowledge of the cause and morbid changes of the disease.

It is not enough to diagnose a *nodular, itching and spreading eruption of the skin,* we must also determine the cause or our prognosis and treatment cannot be correct and rational. Such eruptions are due to various causes and an exact knowledge of them is an important item. The same may be said of affections of internal organs.

A final diagnosis is made either by considering the determined symptoms directly (*direct diagnosis*) or by a *process of exclusion,* i. e., we review in our mind all the diseases in which the symptoms determined occur, or in which some of these symptoms occur, and then we exclude those diseases in the course of which, if present, we usually observe additional symptoms (*differential diagnosis*).

The difficulties encountered in diagnosing internal diseases vary considerably; in some cases a good anamnesis suffices as a basis for making a *definite* diagnosis: epilepsy, parturient paresis. In other cases the experienced practitioner requires but a glance at the patient: tetanus. The rule, however, is never to make a diagnosis until a thorough and careful examination of the patient has been made; but here, too, carefully cultivated powers of observation and extensive experience go a good way. To acquire either of these, of course, requires continued carefully and methodically conducted examinations. The same diseases do not always present the same set of symptoms. Therefore, the more often a disease is seen by the practitioner, the more readily will he recognize it. In the course of one and the same disease the symptoms will change, depending upon whether the onset, acme or latter stages are being observed. The diagnostician should be like the experienced botanist who recognizes a plant in all its stages of vegetation. There will always remain a few cases the symptoms of which are so atypical that an exact diagnosis is impossible.

Not infrequently, however, even the experienced practitioner must content himself with limiting his diagnosis to a statement of the general character of the disease and reserve the privilege of expressing his final opinion (*special diagnosis*) pending further observation and developments. This is particularly the case in the first outbreaks of infectious diseases when localized changes are absent and in many chronic diseases showing few symptoms.

We also distinguish between *a definite, a probable,* and *a possible* diagnosis.

I. Anamnesis.

Full statements on the part of the owner or attendant, procured by cautious questioning, concerning the previous condition of the patient, the beginning and previous course of the disease (*anamnesis*) are of great importance in diagnostics. In fact there are some diseases, like epilepsy, for example, that can as a rule be diagnosed in no other way because it is only in exceptional cases that we have an opportunity to observe a typical epileptic fit.

As far as the veterinarian is concerned the anamnesis is limited to the observation of the immediate surroundings of the animal. In questioning attendants speak to them in a pleasant tone and manner and use words and expressions with which they are familiar; this tends to infuse confidence and the result is that the information thus obtained will be more apt to be reliable.

Any digression in the testimony of informants should be listened to with patience. One should always remember that every anamnesis, from whomsoever it be obtained, is more or less colored by the personal conceptions of the person offering it. This is quite apart from intentional misrepresentations, which are often encountered.

A well drawn up anamnesis speaks for the technical ability of the veterinarian as well as for his knowledge of the etiology of the diseases of our domestic animals which are kept under the most variable conditions.

1. How long has the animal been sick? We may learn by this question whether the disease is an acute or a chronic one, and perhaps also the stage of development

which the disease has reached. Frequently the time given by the owner or attendant is much shorter than the actual duration of the disease.

2. What symptoms has the animal shown? In the beginning? Later on? The objective observation of the owner must be carefully sifted out from his subjective interpretation of them.

3. What, in your opinion, could be the cause of the disease? We cannot search for the causes until we know the symptoms.

Where and under what conditions did the animal get sick? Feed, care, etc., play an important role in the etiology of the internal diseases of animals; therefore the veterinarian must be informed not only as to the kind and character of the feed but also as to soil conditions, water, etc., otherwise he cannot intelligently trace the cause of the disease.

The care and attention animals receive wield a great influence upon the genesis of many diseases. It is rare that the veterinarian can obtain from the attendants reliable data concerning these. He should judge by the surroundings in this regard. The use to which the animal was put when the disease occurred is of value in tracing the cause, for special uses predispose animals to certain diseases.

4. A number of animals affected by the same disease always points to a common cause, viz.: infection or intoxication (*poisoning*). The frequent recurrence of a disease in the same stable points to the existence of a permanent cause.

5. It is of especial importance for the veterinarian to know whether any previous treatment has been resorted to and what effect this may have had. Quacks often administer drenches containing solid particles in suspension; these draughts, instead of taking their usual course, may enter the trachea and thus produce a fatal pneumonia. In removing the contents of the rectum its wall or mucous membrane is

also often injured. In such cases the veterinarian must exercise care and judgment and call the owner's attention to any existing danger.

Although the main points in the anamnesis should be determined before we begin our objective examination, other questions will present themselves in the course of the latter. Thus, when examining the respiratory tract we may inquire whether the animal coughs, and when examining the digestive apparatus inquire as to condition of bowels, frequency of evacuation, etc., in this way gradually completing our examination.

The value of a good anamnesis consists in the fact that not infrequently it is sufficient to base upon it a definite diagnosis, i. e., careful objective observations of the layman may in some instances be substituted for our examination. However, the veterinarian must always be cautious in complying with the oft made request of owners to treat their animals *in absentia.* Although the medicines prescribed under such conditions may do no particular harm, rational treatment thus delayed may prove to be a positive injury.

Sometimes the veterinarian is misled by the anamnesis. This he may guard against by making a careful examination of the patient. When the anamnesis does not conform to the results of the examination, it should be accepted with caution; where the opposite is true, it may be considered reliable.

II. Determining the Status Praesens.

To determine pathological phenomena we resort to all those methods which throw light upon the physical state and functions of the different organs. In doing this we should endeavor to follow a definite plan and not proceed without system. The following methods are generally employed and in the order given:

1. Inspection.

In examining the different parts of the body it is always best that we first regard that which can be observed with the unaided eye. Students are apt to lay their hands upon the patient too soon. Superficial abnormalities are described according to their seat, size, color and other external manifestations; the size and form usually being compared with common objects, unless an exact description is desired when actual measurements are made.

The odor emitted by the se- and excretions and the respirations is also noted.

In designating the seat of visible pathological conditions the exact anatomical region occupied by them should be indicated.

Regions of the Body.

I. Head.

A. Face.

1. Nasal region with dorsum of nose, tip of nose, nasal openings. [Nostrils].
2. Labial region, with upper and lower lips, interlabial space and chin.
3. Buccal region.
4. Infraorbital region.

5. Ocular region.
6. Masseteric region with maxillary articulation.
7. Intermaxillary space.

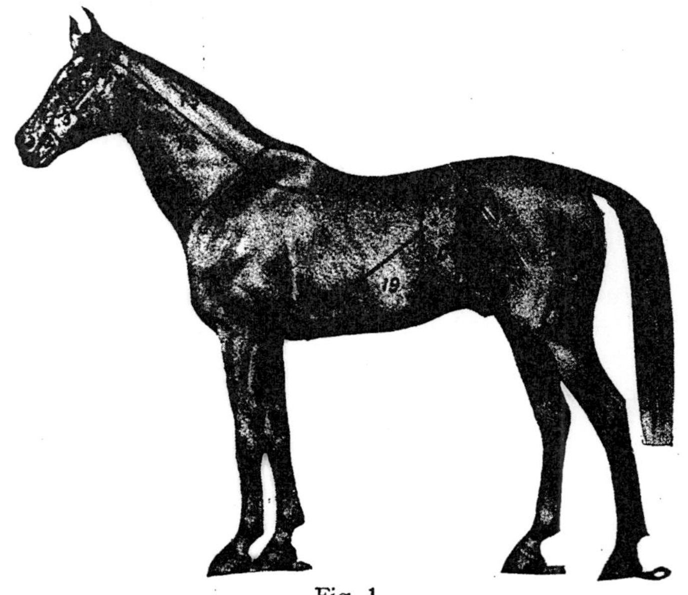

Fig. 1.

B. Forehead.
8. Frontal region.
9. Occipital region with forelock.
10. Temporal region with the temporal fossa, infratemporal groove and auricular region. [Ears].

II. **Neck.**

11. Parotid region, which merges below into the laryngeal region.
12. Tracheal region with jugular groove, at the lower end of which is the supra-clavical fossa.
13. Cervical region with crest and mane.
14. Lateral cervical region, sides of neck.

III. **Chest.**

15. Withers and dorsal region.
16. Lateral pectoral region [side of chest] with scap-

ular region, cardiac region, costal region.

17. Sterinal region.
18. Anterior pectoral region. [Breast].

IV. Abdomen.

19. Epigastric region with xiphoid space.
20. Mesogastric region with umbilical space, iliac region (flank with "hollow of flank") and the lumbar region.
21. Hypogastric region with pubic and inguinal region.

V. Pelvis.

The different divisions of the pelvis are named according to their anatomical parts; the sacral region is called the croup, the external angle of the ilium the "hip," just below the anus the perineal region; the anal region, pubic region and inguinal region.

VI. Extremities.

The different parts of the extremities are designated according to the bones and joints which form their bases. Anterior limb: Shoulder, point of shoulder, arm, elbow, forearm, "knee," cannon, fetlock joint, pastern, coronet, bulbs of heels, hoof. Posterior limb: Thigh, stifle, leg, hock, hind cannon, etc.

2. Palpation.

Palpation consists in feeling the part to be examined with the hand or finger tips. Its object is to gain information through the sense of touch as to the consistency, extent, temperature and sensitiveness of a part, and permit us to recognize abnormalities which do not lie far below the surface. Palpation is of especial importance in taking the pulse. The abdominal viscera can be explored (palpated) through the rectum and the anatomical position, and condition of the contents determined.

From the difference in consistency of the parts palpated, conclusions as to their physical nature may be drawn. The following peculiarities may be distinguished on palpation:

1. A part is *doughy* when it feels soft and accepts finger imprints which it retains for a few moments, when the depressions are again filled. Tissue is of a doughy consistency when infiltrated with serum: (*edema*).

2. A part is *firm* when it is of the consistency of normal liver. According to the part's resistance to the touch it may be firm, tendinous, solid. A cellular infiltration of tissues (*phlegmon*) or the presence of neoplasms made up of cells, will lend to a part a *firm* consistency (connective tissue).

3. A part is *hard* when of the consistency of bone.

4. A part is *fluctuating* when it is soft, elastic and undulates on pressure. Only fluids admit of such a rapid transmission of pressure (pus, blood, lymph, serum). If the tissue surrounding the fluid is not tense, waves are seen to pass over the surface of the swelling (true or soft fluctuations). Soft-elastic (fat) tissue or tissue impregnated with a quantity of fluid may also show fluctuation; this undulating consistency is spoken of as *pseudo-fluctuation*.

5. A part is *emphysematous* when it presents a puffy swelling which crackles and shifts on palpation; it is due to the presence of air or gas in the tissue (*emphysema*).

3. Percussion.

By percussion we understand striking the surface of the animal body so that the parts thus set in vibration emit audible sounds. The "*percussion-sound*" thus produced will differ with the physical condition of the vibrating parts, and these differences are so well marked that definite conclusions can be drawn from them.

Methods of percussion. Percussion can be practiced without the use of instruments [so-called *immediate* percussion] on small animals or large animals thin in flesh. The index or middle finger of the left hand is held firmly against the part to be percussed and struck with the middle finger of the right hand. The striking finger should be held somewhat curved and stiff. The advantage of immediate percussion lies in the facility with which the finger may be placed between the ribs and amid the long hair of some dogs and the wool of sheep. By this method the sense of hearing is further greatly assisted by that of feeling. For the larger animals the sounds obtained from this finger-to-finger method of percussion are not definite enough for practical use.

In the immediate method of percussion, however, the sound can be augmented by employing the percussion hammer to strike the finger which is applied to the part (finger-hammer percussion).

The pleximeter and hammer (plexor) are most commonly used in practice [so-called *mediate* percussion] as they permit not only of gentle percussion but the part to be examined can be struck a heavy blow which sets deep-lying parts into vibration. The pleximeter should be so held that its whole surface is in firm contact with the part be percussed. In thin animals the pleximeter should never be applied across two ribs, but should be made to occupy an intercostal space that the air between it and the body does not modify the sound. The force with which we use the hammer depends upon the thickness of the walls of the part percussed. [In fat animals it is necessary to use more force than in lean ones.]

Usually two or three strokes, not too close together, suffice to bring out clearly the character of the sound. For comparison it is advisable to percuss corresponding parts on each side of the body.

For a better conception of the percussion-sound it is advisable to select a suitable place. A room with closed doors is the best; in rooms filled with furniture, or out of doors the application of percussion is never satisfactory.

As a rule large animals are percussed while standing, though small ones may be placed in a recumbent position upon a table. Although gentle animals may stand quietly during the operation, very nervous horses or stubborn cows sometimes resist. They can generally be quieted by speaking to them in an assuring tone and by omitting all rough usage of the instruments. Dogs and cats may be held by their owners or an attendant.

The Qualities of Percussion-Sounds.

A body can only then produce a sound when it has lost its equilibrium and vibrates by virtue of its elasticity. Two principles form the basis of percussion:

1. Solid, airless parts of the body give forth a flat sound of short duration and little intensity. Such a sound is called *dull*, femoral or *flat*.

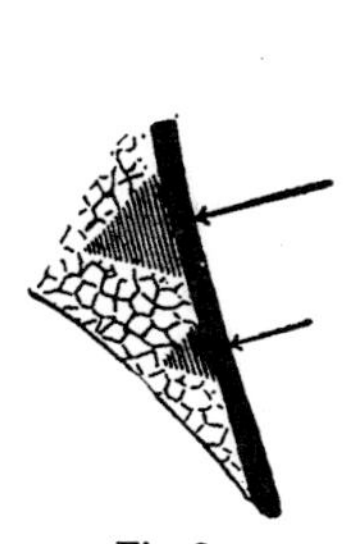

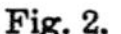

Fig. 2.

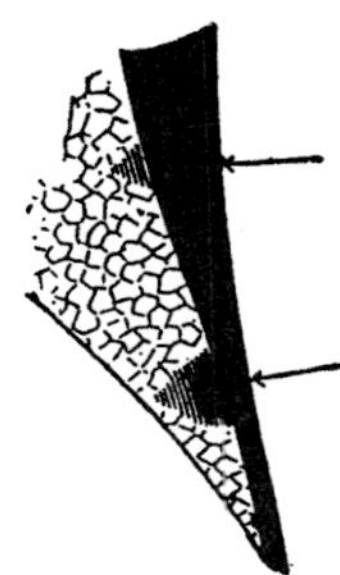

Fig. 3.

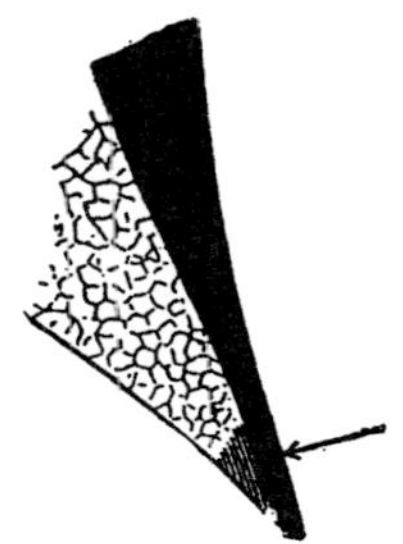

Fig. 4.

2. If an air-containing organ is set in vibration it produces a sound of considerable intensity, duration and tone, the so-called *resonant* sound.

The clearness of the sound depends upon the volume of the air-containing organ which is vibrating.

a. The stronger the percussion the larger is the part which vibrates and the fuller the sound (Fig. 2).

b. The thinner the over-lying tissue of the thoracic wall the more lung tissue will vibrate and the fuller the sound (Fig. 3).

c. If the volume of the air-containing organ is small in itself then the sound is correspondingly less intensive (Fig. 4).

This explains the varying intensity of the sound over different portions of the chest wall when the percussion blows are applied with equal force. The resonant sound gradually merges into the dull femoral as we approach the forward and upper portions.

The resonant sound may be divided into:

1. The *tympanitic* sound which is emitted when the vibrations of the tissue are uniform. It approaches a musical sound and is, therefore, spoken of as a *tympanitic tone.*

2. The *full* sound which is emitted when the vibrations of the tissue are not uniform. It lacks the musical quality of the tympanitic tone and approaches a noise.

The tympanitic tone and the full sound merge into each other gradually. The sound between is called *"over-full"* or *"over-loud."*

The tympanitic tone and the full sound are resonant in character. They may become modified as to clearness until they are absolutely dull (flat). The intermediate stages are *dull resonant* and *dull tympanitic.*

Occurrence of the Different Qualities of Percussion-Sounds.

According to the above classification there are three kinds of percussion-sounds: The *full* (pulmonary resonant), the *tympanitic,* and the *flat.*

1. The *full* sound is found over normal lung, the air in the alveoli, and the lung tissue, and thoracic walls vibrating. When the intestines are so distended with gas that when percussed their walls vibrate with their contents, a full sound is emitted.

2. The *tympanitic* percussion-sound has a varied origin. It is heard:

a. Over cavities containing air which communicate with the outside world, their walls being either firm or yielding: trachea, caverns in the lung communicating with bronchi. The pitch of the sound depends upon the size of the cavern and its communicating opening.

b. Over enclosed air-containing cavities, hence over the stomach and bowels.

c. When air-containing lung tissue is surrounded by solidified portions as occurs in beginning hepatization, edema, atelectasis and tumors of the lung.

3. The *flat* (femoral, dull) sound is heard when percussing over solid tissues which do not contain air. As the most forcible percussion does not produce vibrations at a point more than 7 cm below the surface, dullness can be noted over the normal lung when the chest walls are covered with heavy muscles, fat, or edematous swellings.

An over-loud sound is emitted when the base of the cecum in the horse or the paunch in the ox is percussed, these organs being greatly distended with gas.

The sound is dulled when air-containing parts of limited dimensions are percussed (borders of the lung, and under thick thoracic wall) or if small airless spaces lie amid those containing air (nodular thickenings in the lung).

During the application of percussion we should note the resistance the part offers to the hammer or striking finger. [To understand what is meant by this the student should strike with the plexor some solid object, as a brick wall, and compare it with the feeling experienced when the human chest is percussed.] By placing the index finger on the back of the hammer the resistance can be better appreciated. From the resistance the amount of vibration that can be induced in the underlying parts may be determined, the greater the former the less developed the latter. For this reason solid, airless parts like muscle give a shallow percussion-sound and cause the hammer to suffer a jar when they are struck.

Tactile Percussion.

The combination of palpation and percussion is called *tactile percussion.* Through this method we endeavor to arrive at the physical condition of deep-lying parts by stroking the tissues covering them.

Method. The wrist and fingers should be held slightly flexed and fixed. The parts to be examined should be pressed firmly with the finger tips, exerting an interrupted stroke. After such a stroke the fingers should be allowed to dwell for a moment to note the recoil of the underlying tissue the consistency of which we wish to determine. In practicing this form of percussion bear in mind that the deeper rather than the shallower tissues are to be felt.

Tactile percussion may also be practiced with the plexor and pleximeter, the index finger being rested upon the back of the hammer. It is usually better, however, to employ hammer-to-finger or finger-to-finger percussion.

The thickness of the over-lying fat or muscular layers does not seriously interfere in this form of percussion. Through practice we learn to select the factors of importance to form an opinion. Deep-lying diseased conditions do not present through tactile percussion specific symptoms, but we may thus obtain valuable information in regard to the boundaries and consistency of otherwise unavailable organs or parts. Tactile percussion simply supplements and completes palpation and ordinary percussion.

Determining the Boundaries of an Organ from the Percussion-Sound.

The boundary of an organ can be determined by percussion only when the organ lies superficially and emits a percussion-sound which differs from that of its neighborhood. For this reason the boundary of the heart against the lung or the lung against the bowels may be defined by percussion.

4. Auscultation.

By *auscultation,* applying the ear to a part, we seek to obtain information, through the sense of hearing, as to the physical state or condition of deep-lying organs. For this reason auscultation is practiced upon the heart, lungs and gastro-intestinal tract.

In human medicine auscultation is usually practiced with the help of instruments (*mediate auscultation*), the so called stethoscope, etc., being employed. [In veterinary medicine, however, the use of such instruments is very limited, the heavy hair coat materially interfering with and so modifying the sounds that false conclusions may be drawn. To a limited extent the phonendoscope is useful in auscultating heart sounds, but the hairs over the cardiac region should first be thoroughly moistened or oiled.]

By simply applying the ear firmly to the part, better results can be obtained than by the use of instruments. In case the skin is dirty, blistered, or the animal is lousy, a towel can be placed between it and the ear. To guard against being bitten or kicked an attendant should hold the patient by the head. In large stables containing a good many animals the noises they produce may interfere with auscultation; if it is essential to diagnosis or prognosis, the patient should be examined in some quieter place.

A. The General Part of the Examination.

I. Signalment.

By the *Signalment* is meant a *description of the patient* for identification by peculiar marks or characteristics. For forensic purposes and special cases the proper taking of the signalment is of great importance. It is further of some value in a diagnostic sense and is sometimes taken into consideration therapeutically.

It includes:

I. **Kind of animal.** Many diseases are peculiar to certain genera while they do not occur in others. This is especially true of the infectious diseases as, for instance, the horse suffers from strangles, and glanders; the ox from contagious pleuropneumonia (lung plague), malignant head catarrh, and swine from hog cholera and swine plague. There are also special sporadic diseases which owe their origin to the peculiar anatomical or physical make-up of a genus. As examples, may be mentioned traumatic pericarditis of the ox; ruptures of the stomach and roaring in the horse.

II. **Sex.** Diseases of the sexual organs are not common in animals, but sex is of influence in the appearance of some diseases. In stallions inguinal hernias which cause symptoms simulating colic occur; mares during the period of heat may act as if they were suffering from some brain disease (act like *dummies*) or may balk or show obstinacy when at work. In the ox urethral calculi are not uncommon. The condition of pregnancy is as of great importance from the diagnostic as from the therapeutical standpoint, because this condition may induce physiological symptoms that would be considered pathological in non-pregnant animals. In pregnant animals caution is demanded in the choice of drugs.

III. Color and white markings. For diagnosis the color and markings are of less importance. White horses frequently suffer from melanotic tumors that are either superficial or located in internal organs. White areas are more predisposed to exanthemas, sunburn and "scratches."

IV. Age. Many diseases occur either exclusively or generally in youth. Rachitis, diseases of the navel, strangles in colts, scours in calves and distemper in puppies are examples. In old individuals diseases due to the animal's use are more frequent as are also chronic diseases of organs (dummies, heaves).

The age is also of influence upon the prognosis in as much as healing, all things else being equal, is more to be hoped for in the young individual than in the old one. In old animals where the prognosis is a doubtful one all treatment is frequently omitted on economic grounds.

V. Size. Size is of importance in posology only.

VI. Breed. In well bred animals the reaction against the encroachment of disease is more energetic and the symptoms are more pronounced. Certain breeds are more able to withstand infectious and sporadic diseases than others, this must be considered in making a prognosis. Breed is also taken into consideration in the treatment of diseases. Woll bred, fine skinned, sensitive horses yield to the action of certain drugs more readily than those of the opposite type. This is especially true where outward applications (turpentine blisters) are to be made.

2. Habitus.

By the term *habitus* we mean the general or external aspect or characteristic appearance of the patient, which is determined by its physical attitude, condition, conformation and temperament. It offers a convenient aid in diagnosis, one that can be readily observed and that, in many respects, is of great importance. Not infrequently a diagnostic conclusion in a clinical case is reached largely through the impression the patient makes upon us by its *habitus.*

Obvious physiological abnormalities are sometimes of themselves an index to the character of the disease. However, one should guard against reaching hasty conclusions from the first impressions of the patient, to the neglect of a thorough examination.

1. *Attitude of the patient.* Healthy horses as a rule remain standing during the day, or if lying down they immediately rise to their feet at the approach of a stranger. They will frequently lie flat on the side with feet extended, provided the halter strap is long enough and the stall of sufficient width.

Healthy cattle lie down often during the day, especially just after feeding, and they are not so prone to rise when approached. They seldom lie flat on the side, but in *sternal decubitus* the limbs folded under them.

Healthy sheep jump up when approached and usually run away.

The attitude of sick animals whether standing, walking or lying down is often of value in diagnosis.

Standing attitudes assumed during disease. The head is held *stiffly* and *extended* in pharyngitis, cerebro-spinal meningitis, muscular rheumatism, malignant head catarrh of the ox, and in acute encephalitis of sheep and goats.

Very sick animals usually hold the *head down,* and assume a *relaxed languid* attitude, the ears drooping; horses rest their feet alternately.

Cows suffering from severe vaginitis stand with *arched back,* tail held high, and legs spread apart. They do not "stand over" readily in the stable, and if driven stop repeatedly to urinate.

A *stiff, quiet* attitude avoiding moving as much as possible, is characteristic of very painful affections in the chest or abdominal walls (pleurodynia, pleuritis, peritonitis). Stallions suffering from incarcerated inguinal hernia and oxen with peritoneal hernia (gut tie) stand with the hind leg of the affected side held backward and outward.

Unphysiological attitudes. Animals afflicted with brain troubles (acute or sub-acute encephalitis, dummies) very often assume unnatural attitudes. Horses stand obliquely in the stall, the head in a corner, resting against the wall or sunk under the feed box. The limbs are drawn well up under the abdomen, and not infrequently one leg is placed in a very unphysiological position, perhaps crossing its fellow of the opposite side. Dummies stand unusually quiet and seem oblivious of their surroundings. They move without energy, and are backed with the utmost difficulty. (See under "Central Nervous System," "Examination of Dummies").

In acute brain diseases the horse does not continuously assume these attitudes but only at times.

Continued standing is observed in:

a. Old, worn-out horses.

b. Pneumonia and Pleuritis. As a rule if the animals lie down in these diseases it is on the diseased side, and for the following reasons: because the slight pressure of the ground against the body ameliorates the pain, and the pleuritic exudate (the effusion in the chest) does not encroach so much upon the heart and the still healthy lung. The respirations are always more difficult when the animal is lying down. [In peritonitis resulting from castration horses very commonly remain standing; when forced to move they do so with hind legs held in abduction, advancing very stiffly].

c. Severe Dyspnea. The *head is held extended* to allow the air the easiest possible access to the lungs, thus facilitating inspiration.

d. Horses suffering from acute diseases of the brain.

e. Horses suffering from Tetanus. The stand with legs braced *like a saw horse,* the *head somewhat extended* and *held high,* the *back held rigid.* It is very difficult for them to step sideways. The facial expression is anxious, the *mem-*

brana nictitans appearing plainly before the eye; the tail is carried high and stiff, and the gait inflexible and laborious.

Restless Standing. Most commonly seen in horses suffering from colic and acute brain diseases. The former are restless, lie down, roll, and get right up again. In many cases it is only with difficulty that they can be kept on their feet; when down it may be equally hard to drive them up. They often look at the flanks, paw, strike the belly with the hind feet, switch the tail, and stretch as if to urinate without voiding urine. At times they sit up like a dog.

Like symptoms but of shorter duration are observed in the ox suffering from invagination of the intestines, torsion of the uterus in cows and from urethral stones and peritoneal hernia in steers.

Horses with acute brain disease show at times rabiform symptoms, plunging, rearing and breaking loose. When not tied they keep forging ahead or continue aimlessly walking in a circle.

Restless, anxious moving about is seen in many cases of severe dyspnea.

Gait. A labored, slow, exhausted, wobbling gait is noted in severe febrile diseases. It is especially marked in influenza of the horse. In tetanus, muscular rheumatism and purpura hemorrhagica the gait is stiff. Lameness of one or more limbs is seen in foot and mouth disease and pyemia (pyemic arthritis). The gait is unphysiological in acute and chronic hydrocephalus. In the trotter disease of sheep the patient does not walk but goes at a stiff trot. The crackling of joints is heard especially in equine influenza.

Lying postures assumed during Disease. Animals found lying down and that can not be made to rise should be examined very carefully. In them the examination is always difficult. We should first try to drive them up by speaking to them in a sharp tone of voice and assisting them by mechanical means. It is important to determine whether they are really unable to rise or whether they are obstinate and will not rise (malingerers).

If the animals have lain for a long time on one side, it is advisable to turn them over before attempting to drive them up. The same should be done when after a fruitless effort to get an animal onto its feet, it falls back again to the ground and we make a second attempt to make it stand.

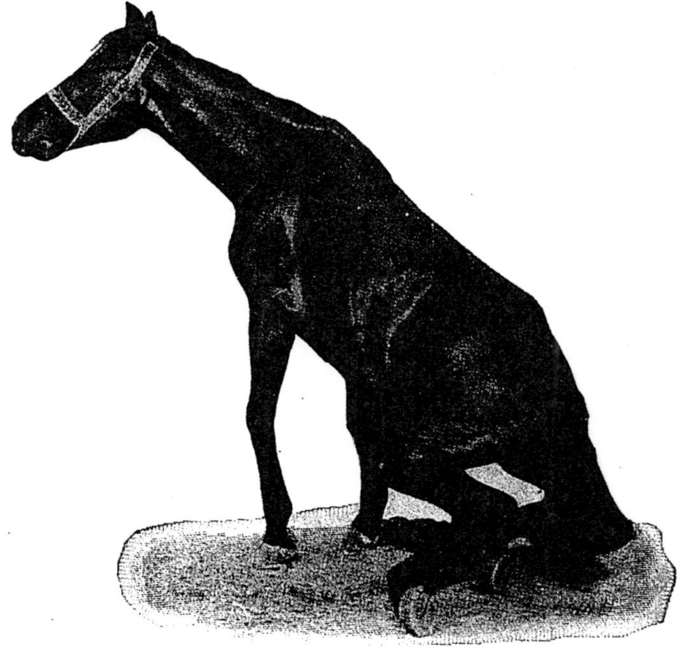

Fig. 5—Horse with Azoturia.

To bring recumbent horses to their feet it is expedient, after placing them on the sternum, to pass the end of a long halter rope through a convenient ring in the wall, and keep it pulled taut; the hind legs should be doubled under the body in a natural position and the fore ones extended in front. By speaking to the animal, striking it over the ears and nose, and lifting by the tail, we may assist it to regain its feet. When this method fails, a sling should be placed under the body and the animal raised with block and tackle.

The ox is often hard to induce to stand up after it has been down for a time. It may be able to get up, but through obstinacy will not do so. Whipping and beating in such cases is usually of no avail; yelling in the animal's ear, setting a dog on it or tieing its nose shut may be tried. [By placing a rope around the body so that it passes beneath the brisket in front and the ischii behind, we have improvised a handle by which several persons can lift the malingerer to its feet.]

Animals may be unable to arise:

a. **In Tetanus.** Horses suffering from tetanus, if down, are as a rule unable to stand up without help, as the spasmodic contractions of the extensors of the limbs prevent it. When recumbent, the upper pair of legs do not come in contact with the ground. The animals are very restless and bedewed with sweat.

Fig. 5a.

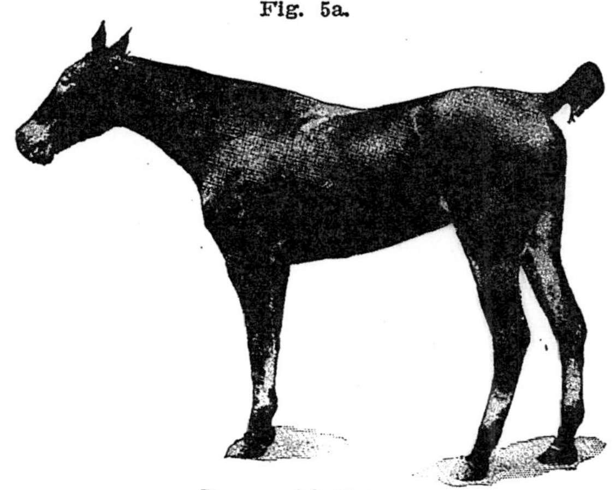

Horse with Tetanus.

b. **In Azoturia.** Horses suffering from acute azoturia make vain efforts to stand. They are sometimes only partially successful, the fore part of the body being raised and supported by the front legs, but the hind limbs are unable to bear their share of the weight, breaking down under it.

c. **In Spinal paralysis** from Fractures of Vertebrae. The patients lose control of the hind parts which are no longer sensible to pain [pin pricks]. Sometimes, however, reflex spinal convulsions attend "broken back." Dogs with paralyzed hind parts usually sit sideways, the legs directed away from the body.

d. **Ante- and Post-partum Paresis.** Occurs in cows before or after calving. The animals seem to be in comparatively good health, have a good appetite, but can not regain their feet. There are no further symptoms of disease or injury. They often lie stretched out on the side. [Prognosis is favorable.]

e. **Milk Fever** (parturient paresis). The cow lies in a comatose condition on the left side as if in profound sleep, the head resting against the right chest. If the head be lifted

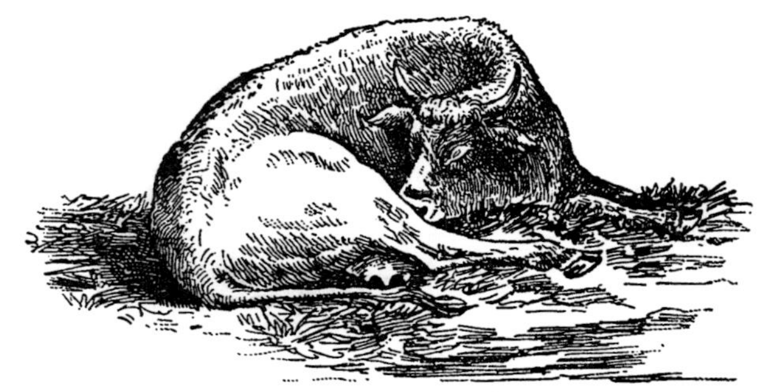

Fig. 6.—Cow with Parturient Paresis.

it drops back again to its former position as soon as released. Sensitiveness and temperature of the whole body are diminished.

f. **Cramp of the Neck** (cerebro-spinal meningitis). After showing symptoms of stiff, wry neck, while standing, paralysis follows. The patients lie flat on the side with the head drawn backward, the body convulsed with spasms.

Old, worn out horses are hard to get upon their feet once they have lain or fallen down. When animals are suffering from severe pain in the legs and feet (founder) or when lying on an injured limb (fracture), they can as a rule rise only with the greatest difficulty. Colic patients, when down, generally do not get up promptly.

Inspection of Herds. In examining groups or entire herds of animals, one should observe the behavior of each individual. The inspection may be conducted in the stable or better in the open, without undue excitement, and any animal showing symptoms carefully noted. Sick animals are recognized by their attitude, movements, depressed appearance, lack of appetite, etc. After such a preliminary survey of the group or herd suspected individuals may be separately scrutinized.

II. Condition. The condition of the animal is recognized principally by the rotundity and fullness of development of the body. Cold blooded horses usually have well rounded forms because the muscles are of large size and surrounded by well developed fat deposits. The condition as to flesh is influenced by the quantity and quality of the food and the use and purpose for which the animal is intended and fed. Continued hard work reduces the fullness of the body outline, causing the conformation to appear angular.

When the digestive tract is affected with disease whether local or general, the condition of the animal becomes reduced. A gradual but continual loss of condition, notwithstanding that the appetite and food are good, always points to chronic disease, but not necessarily to disease of the digestive tract. When the digestive tract becomes diseased the appetite is impaired.

Depending upon the use and purpose of the animal we distinguish the following kinds of condition: *Prime, very good, tolerably good, fair* and *bad.* A gradual, progressive general emaciation is called *Cachexia.* Rapid emaciation appears in purpura hemorrhagica and in severe infectious diseases. Excessive corpulency (obesity) is common in bulls and dogs.

If the patient's condition as to flesh is of importance to consider, it is well to note the things by which condition is determined, such as the size of the muscles, thickness of the crest, fat over the ribs, number of ribs visible, prominence of the spines of the dorsal vertebrae, etc. The best way to determine whether the patient is gaining or losing in condition is to weigh it, which should be done each morning, preferably before feeding.

Of importance in diagnosis is the difference between *thinness* and *emaciation.* Thinness is physiological and is peculiar to certain breeds of animals. The thin (lean) animal may feel well, show good appetite, smooth, lustrous hair coat, and render efficient service (large milk flow). Emaciation, on the other hand, is a condition due to disease, starvation or old age. If for any reason the digestive tract can not perform its functions emaciation results. Rapid emaciation occurs in purpura hemorrhagica and in all severe infectious diseases. Emaciated animals show a dull, erect hair coat, leathery, dry skin, are languid and present varied disease symptoms.

III. Conformation. It is advisable to classify horses according to their use into heavy and light draft, carriage and saddle horses. The classification is based upon the animal's conformation. To judge of the conformation correctly we should take into consideration the depth of the body, breadth, depth of chest, curvature of the ribs, length of back, depth of flank, breadth of pelvis, strength and angulation of the joints, and the attitude of the limbs when standing naturally.

Accordingly, we distinguish between a strong and weak, heavy and light boned, well muscled and poorly muscled conformation.

Horses with flat, small chests possess poor staying qualities, the lungs correlatively being small. Horses with flat, not well sprung ribs, tucked up abdomens and long legs, are as a rule poor feeders. As such animals show continually poor appetite for food, the bowels are not kept well filled, hence the body appears deficient in depth. Hearty horses, good feeders, show on the other hand, better developed abdomens, the bowels being distended by the large quantities of food they contain. The more voluminous the food, the greater the circumference of the belly. [The abdominal circumference is further increased in pregnancy and in diseases causing exudates to accumulate in the abdominal cavity, *ascites*].

Animals with curvature of the spine, abnormal bending of the leg bones or diffuse enlargements of joints suffer or have suffered from constitutional bone diseases in youth (rachitis). Calves with broad, beefy hind parts and wide loins, suffer from pelvic distortion, grow slowly and should not be used for breeding ("Doppellender").

IV. Temperament. By temperament we mean the mental attitude the animal assumes toward impressions perceived through the medium of the organs of sense. An animal's knowledge of what is going on about it is obtained through the instrumentality of the bodily senses of sight, hearing, smell, and touch. We distinguish between a *lively* and a *phlegmatic* temperament, comparing the power of quick perception with its opposite slow comprehension. Too much tendency in either direction will affect the usefulness of an animal.

Animals of fiery disposition often show temper by being *stubborn, vicious, balky,* or they are very *nervous, anxious, easily frightened,* which reduces their economic value. Young animals, especially horses, are often restless and like to play.

Animals of a very phlegmatic temperament may be so slow to move as to impair their usefulness.

The sort of temperament possessed by an animal is shown by its external appearance. The countenance, expression of the eye, play of the ears, and quickness of movement form sources from which the temperament and disposition may be judged. The facial expression and eye give information as to the mental condition.

Blind horses are often scary; they employ the sense of hearing, moving the ears in a lively manner to take the place of the lost sense of sight, at the same time holding the head still. This may cause us at first sight to suspect that the animal is suffering from a brain disease. Old horses are not so sensitive to outside impressions as colts. Some colts, however, are little observing of their surroundings, appearing dull, stupid and lazy, without suffering from disease. Great fatigue produces temporary mental depression in individuals.

Febrile diseases affect the temperament, making the animal affected sluggish in its movements. In animals of fiery temperament this is not so noticeable.

In animals suffering from severe, serious diseases, the temperament can become so changed that vices, such as cribbing, biting, kicking, etc., are no longer indulged in. The countenance appears blank, expressionless, staring, eyes sunken, locomotion slow and unsteady. A few hours before the fatal termination of a disease, the normal *tonus* of the tissues is lost, the muscles relax, especially those of the face, forming the so-called Hippocratic countenance (*facies Hippocratica*), one of the symptoms of approaching death.

Diseases Which Are Characterized Particularly by Change in Habitus.

Tetanus. See pages 37 and 220.

Colic is a complex of symptoms in the horse characterized by abdominal pain and suppressed peristalsis. It is due to some affection of the stomach or bowels. For the symptoms in regard to manner in which pain is shown, see page 35. Further symptoms are sweating, congested, "muddy" conjunctiva, accelerated pulse, dyspnea, anorexia, suppressed peristalsis, obstipation. The cause which lies at the bottom of these clinical phenomena can be determined only by careful examination of the abdomen. (See this.)

Azoturia is an acute auto-intoxication in the horse characterized principally by a peculiar severe parenchymatous inflammation and paralysis of the muscles and complicated by hemoglobinemia and acute nephritis. It appears suddenly under symptoms of paralysis of one or both hind limbs, inability to stand, restlessness and sweating. Croup muscles tense, hemoglobinemia, hematuria. No fever, mind clear, dyspnea, appetite retained. When standing knuckle in joints of affected limb; make ineffectual efforts to regain feet; hind limbs unable to support body.

Polyarthritis (articular rheumatism). Febrile infectious disease with inflammation of usually several joints. Without apparent external cause there appear suddenly hot and painful swellings of joints. Patients remain lying; high temperature, no appetite, cease ruminating. Most common in ox; rare in horse.

Muscular rheumatism (myositis rheumatica). Peculiar inflammation of individual muscles or groups of muscles. Characterized by wandering, periodical pains. Mostly confined to limbs and back; head rarely affected. Temperature not high. Not infrequently complicates other diseases, especially those due to refrigeration. Most common in horse, dog and swine.

Cerebro-spinal meningitis (cramp of the neck). Probably infectious. Symptoms vary. Delirium, spasms of the muscles of the head, neck and limbs. High fever; dysphagia. Patients remain lying with head drawn back (opisthotonus).

Parturient paresis (milk fever). See page 38.

Rachitis and osteomalacia. Both of these diseases are characterized by the bones being deficient in lime salts. Such bones

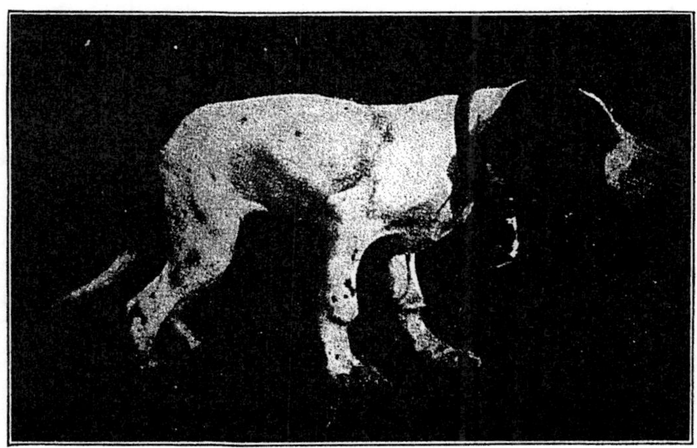

Fig. 7.—Rachitic Dog.

possess little power of sustaining weight, hence they suffer change in form when weight of the body must be borne by them.

a. **Rachitis** appears only in young animals, mostly in pigs and puppies. Pathologically the disease may be considered to be a remaining softness of the bones, the epiphyses becoming enlarged, the diaphyses bent. An upward curvature of the spine ⌒ is called kyphosis, a downward ⌣ lordosis, a lateral) scoliosis. Animals suffering from rachitis remain lying a great deal, find trouble in regaining their feet, and locomotion is difficult.

b. **Osteomalacia.** Fragility of the bones is seen only in adult animals (cattle). The animals lie down continually, are weak, eat but little, and become thin in flesh. The bones of the extremities become brittle; spontaneous fractures, decubitus, and death ensue.

3. The Skin.

The condition of the skin indicates the state of health. The condition of the skin is affected not only in local diseases of that organ, but in many maladies of a general nature, involving internal viscera. An examination of the integument, therefore, is of importance to diagnosis. The skin is examined by inspection and palpation; in local diseases the microscope is employed. An examination of the skin includes the following:

I. Condition of the hair coat. In horses and cattle in good condition the hair is usually *short, fine, glossy,* and lies smoothly. Horses running on pasture or kept in unsanitary stables, show a *long, lusterless, rough, bristling,* hair coat. If the condition of the hair coat is bad, notwithstanding good care and shelter, it may be assumed that the animal is suffering from ill health. The appearance of the hair coat is influenced mostly by chronic diseases. Temporarily the hairs may become erect when the animal is carrying increased temperature (chill) or from the effects of cold air or water.

In birds with fever the feathers appear ruffled, especially those of the neck which stand erect.

In long haired animals the hair coat should lie closely matted and the hairs have the same general direction. A *tufting* of the wool of sheep is indicative of skin disease (scabies).

Shedding of the hair. In horses and cattle a partial shedding of the hair occurs normally each fall and spring. In the fall the long, soft winter coat appears; this is shed the following spring. [Animals kept blanketed in warm stables retain a short hair coat throughout the winter.] Good care and proper food hasten the shedding of the hair, contrary conditions tend to postpone it. When the winter coat is retained during the summer months, it indicates usually chronic disease of nutrition.

When horses which have been poorly kept pass into good hands and receive nourishing food and good attention, an unusually early shedding of the winter coat follows.

Loss of Hair. A loss of hair over the whole or a large part of the body (*alopecia*) sometimes quickly follows the recovery of an animal from a severe infectious disease (contagious pleuropneumonia of the horse). A gradual loss of coat accompanies chronic, cachectic diseases in sheep and dogs. In chronic diseases affecting nutrition the hairs become loose, and may be easily removed by pulling or rubbing. Horses clipped late in the season (November, December) grow short winter coats; when these are shed the following spring, the skin is left partially denuded of hair, giving the animal a half-naked appearance.

Where the hairs fall out in patches, and lesions are found in the skin, a disease of the integument is present.

II. Sweat secretion. The skin is kept continually moist by the secretions of the sweat glands. In healthy animals at rest the supply of secretion is just sufficient to keep pace with the loss by evaporation, so that the skin does not feel wet but soft and pliable. The skin's moisture is increased by exercise, high atmospheric temperatures and nervous excitement. Sweating does not become visible in swine, sheep, dogs, and cats.

In disease a more or less profuse outbreak of sweat (*hyperidrosis*) appears:—

1. In severe dyspnea, where it is compensatory, assisting the lungs to throw off effete matter; stenosis of the anterior respiratory passages, diffuse pneumonias, pulmonary emphysemas, and organic heart diseases.

2. In painful maladies: founder, colic, enteritis.

3. In diseases painfully affecting the muscles: tetanus, epilepsy, azoturia, cerebro-spinal meningitis.

4. In severe infectious diseases, septicemia, pyemia.

5. When an animal is much weakened from acute or chronic disease.

Normally, perspiration is accompanied by a hyperemia of the whole skin (*"hot sweat"*). If this congestion is absent the sweat being excreted upon a cold skin surface, *"cold sweat"* is spoken of, a condition to be judged unfavorably from a prognostic standpoint.

Local sweating (*hyperidrosis localis*), or sweat appearing on only one side of the body (*hemidrosis*) is seen at times to accompany diseases of the nervous system.

A decrease in sweat secretion (*hyphidrosis*) can be so well developed that the skin feels dry (*anidrosis*). This condition can best be appreciated on the muzzle of the ox, the snout of the hog, or the nose-tip of the dog. These parts in healthy animals are moist and nearly cold. During high fever, severe diarrhea, diabetes insipidus (*polyuria*), hyphidrosis is a common attending symptom. In severe diseases where life is threatened, the nose feels cold and dry.

III. Swellings in, and immediately under, the skin. Diffuse or multiple swellings appearing in or immediately under the skin are of great importance as an aid to the diagnosis of internal diseases which they accompany.

Tumefactions of the skin attend the following morbid processes:

Edema of the skin and subcutis (*anasarca*) is an abnormal accumulation of serum in the connective tissue. It is produced by a transudation of fluid (liquor sanguinis) from the blood into the intercellular spaces. The lymph spaces being clogged prevents the escape of the fluid. Edematous swellings are *doughy* on palpation and retain finger imprints.

Edema can be due to:

a. Continued venous congestion, the free circulation of the blood being interrupted (*dropsy from stasis*). In such cases a dropsical swelling appears in pendent portions of the body, removed from the heart. The prepuce, in front of the mammæ, ventrally along the abdomen and thorax, hind limbs, brisket and throat are the favorite seats of these enlargements which are neither painful nor hot. Any morbid condition which interferes with the free flow of the blood through the veins, leading to a stagnation in these vessels, tends always to produce edematous swellings. They attend organic heart troubles, chronic pleuritis, pericarditis, and traumatic pericarditis of the ox.

b. A watery condition of the blood (*hydremia*) with which occurs an abnormal porosity of the blood vessels, and a subsequent transudation into the tissues. The edema of hydremia shows neither increased warmth nor pain. Contrary to edema due to venous congestion (stasis), the infiltrated tissue is usually not reddened but pale, anemic. Dropsies due to hydremia are noted under the jaws of sheep afflicted with animal parasites, [the lung and stomach worms, *Str. contortus, Str. filaria;* liver flukes, *Dist. hepaticum,* being the most common]. Leucemia and anemia are frequently attended with skin dropsies.

c. Inflammatory edema (collateral edema) also produces swellings of the skin, but this is usually local. It is characterized by pain and increased warmth. In one form of anthrax appears a circumscribed, hot, hard, painful tumor on the neck, head, or body—the malignant carbuncle.

In some of the infectious diseases a more or less diffuse, or a multiple inflammatory edema, becomes manifest; in influenza of the horse the eyelids, scrotum and limbs swell; in purpura hemorrhagica multiple, later diffuse tumefactions occur on the head, prepuce, lower abdomen, and limbs. [Leg swellings in purpura are characterized by their abrupt, bolster-like, termination]. A local, hot, edematous swelling often betrays the presence of deep-lying inflammation—pus, and is therefore important in diagnosis. In strangles of horses suppuration in unavailable lymph glands is determined by the accompanying edema of the skin in the region of the throat; in glanders it occurs about the farcy bud; in traumatic peritonitis of cattle a hot, doughy swelling appears in the hypochondrium.

Emphysema of the skin. Emphysema of the skin signifies the presence of air in the subcutaneous tissue. Such swellings *crackle* on palpation and are usually *well de-*

fined. The contained air can be temporarily displaced by applying pressure to parts of the swelling, but as soon as the pressure is released the space caused by it refills.

Emphysema originating spontaneously is infrequent. It is mostly due to the formation of gas in decomposing blood extravasates or retained abscesses (*emph. septicum*). Spontaneous emphysema is pathognomonic of *black leg,* where it appears upon the back, neck, and muscular portions of the legs.

Emphysema occurs also from the aspiration of air from without into the subcutis. The air may enter through a wound in the skin, or may come from some air-containing internal organ.

In the first case the air is sucked or pumped into the subcutis through skin wounds which continually shift position during locomotion. Wounds in the neighborhood of the elbow, therefore, produce emphysema of the shoulder and neck. It is a common practice to treat atrophies of superficial muscles ("sweeny") by inflating the overlying skin with air artificially introduced by a bicycle pump or pipe stem]. In the second case the emphysema of the skin has its origin from an internal organ, usually the lung, the alveoli of which are ruptured (*interstitial pulmonary emphysema*). The course followed by the air is as follows: It passes from the ruptured alveoli into the subpleural connective tissue, making its way to the mediastinum, between which folds it continues to the upper part of the thorax, then following the course of the trachea, large blood vessels and esophagus, it escapes from the pectoral cavity through its anterior aperture into the subcutaneous and intermuscular tissues. Rupture of the pulmonary alveoli may result from a destruction of the lung tissue by pus or putrefaction (gangrene). Rib fractures involving the lung, great intra-thoracic pressure from violent coughing, continued bellowing, forced contraction (straining) of the abdominal muscles in bowel, bladder and uterine troubles, may be at the bottom of emphysema of the integument.

Sometimes after rumenotomy or trocaring, gas passes from the paunch through the muscular wound into the subcutaneous tissue. The skin wound having shifted position, the escape of the gas to the surface is prevented, hence it collects in the loose connective tissue along the back.

IV. Color of the skin. The hair and pigment prevent us from seeing that color of the skin which is caused by the blood and other physiological fluids flowing through it. With the exception of the horse, nearly all white-coated animals have non-pigmented skins: [Horses having white or grey hair coats show pigmented skins, the white-born (albino) horses forming an exception. The parts of the skin which show white markings (legs, forehead) are as a rule not colored.]

Chronic discharges from natural openings (the eye, nose, vulva) cause a loss of pigment from the portions of the skin over which they flow.

An injection (reddening) of the skin is only of diagnostic importance when not produced by local diseases of the integument. A diffuse reddening of the skin, namely of the abdomen, neck and between the thighs, is seen in swine erysipelas (*Rothlauf*). Red spots, often angular in shape, accompanied by swelling of the skin, appearing usually over the neck and along the back, are seen in urticaria and in mild cases of erysipelas in swine.

The skin becomes bluish red (cyanotic) when the blood is heavily charged with carbonic acid gas. It is seen in diseases causing swelling of the glottis, heart diseases, congestion and edema of the lungs, and in overdriven sheep or swine during hot weather.

A sharply defined, highly red or dark red discoloration of the ears appears in chronic swine erysipelas (*Rothlauf*) and in peracute hog cholera. In the latter the temperature may be normal or subnormal.

Yellow (icteric) discoloration and paleness of the skin will be considered under "Examination of the Conjunctiva." See page 59.)

V. Condition of the skin. The skin of a healthy animal feels *pliable* and *elastic,* and is movable upon its underlying tissues. If a fold of it be drawn out between the fingers, it soon regains its former place when released.

Where the animal is poorly nourished, out of condition, or emaciated from wasting disease, the skin feels *hard* and *leather-like* (sclerosis, induration). [If the subcutis has also lost its elasticity, and the skin adheres closely to the underlying parts, and cannot readily be drawn out in folds, it causes a condition that is commonly termed "hide boundness"].

In the hide bound animal the epidermis is dry and tough, the outer epidermal layer becomes loose and may be easily removed.

The skin is thus coated with a thick layer of scales and the hair filled with dandruff.

The exhalations of the skin sometimes have a penetrating *urinous* odor, noted not infrequently from bladder rupture, the contents of the organ being poured into the abdominal cavity. This condition is noted following urethral calculi in the ox.

Diseases of the Skin.

The following terms are most commonly employed to denominate the phenomena of skin lesions:

1. Spots (*maculae*) are well circumscribed abnormal colorations of the skin.

2. Papules (*papulae*) are small cutaneous elevations of solid consistency varying in size from that of a pin head to that of a small pea.

3. Vesicles (*vesiculae*) are elevations of the outer epidermal layer due to the accumulation of fluid beneath. They vary from the size of a millet-seed to that of a pea.

4. Blisters (*bullae*) are large vesicles.

5. Pustules (*pustulae*) are vesicles containing pus, and are therefore colored yellow.

6. Ulcers (*ulcera*) are suppurating wound surfaces which result from necrosis of tissue.

7. Scales (*squamae*) are epidermic lamellae which have become detached from the skin's surface.

8. Scabs, or crusts, are dried masses of exudate upon the surface of the integument.

9. Hives (urticaria, nettle rash) are due to swellings of the papillary bodies, producing well-defined evanescent rounded elevations, resembling welts raised by a whip.

I. Non-parasitic Skin Diseases.

1. **Alopecia** (baldness) is a loss of hair due to some disturbance in the skin's nutrition. It may not be attended by lesion.

2. **Blood sweating** (*hematidrosis*) is the spontaneous appearance of blood upon the apparently intact surface of the integument. It is peculiar to Hungarian and Oriental horses.

3. **Prurigo** is a papular eruption accompanied by intense itching. Biting and rubbing induce additional lesions.

4. **Summer surfeit** (*acne simplex*) is a nodular eruption occurring usually over the neck and shoulders, leading to a loss of hair. [It is seen mostly during the hot months. This condition is often erroneously attributed to some "disorder of the blood." Its chief cause is neglect of proper grooming and care of the skin of horses.]

5. **Fagopyrism** is an acute, diffuse, itchy inflammation of the non-pigmented skin of the head, due to grazing on growing buckwheat in bright sunshine. Brain symptoms sometimes complicate the disease.

6. **Eczema.** In a general way the term eczema designates an exudative dermatitis. It has much in common with the catarrhs of mucous membranes, and like the latter can pass through the varied stages of erythema with desquamation, papule, vesicle and pustule formation and finally squammae. It is very common in dogs, appearing along the back and tail.

7. **Foot eczema,** produced by potato residue, swill and brewer grain feeding, is a vesicular eczema occurring on the hind legs of the ox. The vesicles rupture soon after formation and their contents dry to thick yellow scabs. The hair of the affected parts stands erect and part of it falls out. In most instances the eczema reaches no higher up the legs than the hock, but may spread to the body or involve the anterior limbs.

II. Skin Diseases Due to Animal Parasites.

The common skin parasites are:

1. **Lice or Pediculidae** (Haematopinus asini, eurysternus, urius, etc.)

2. **Bird lice or Mallophaga** (Trichodectes equi, scalaria, etc.)*

3. **Louse flies or Hippoboscidae** (Hippobosca equina, Melophagus ovis).

4. **Ticks or Ixodidae** (Boophilus bovis) *Texas cattle tick.*

5. **Fleas or Siphonaptera** (Ceratopsyllus serraticeps of dog, Pulex irritans of man).

6. **Bird ticks or Gamasidae** (Dermanyssus avium, D. gallinae).

7. **Mites or Acarina** (Chorioptes, symbiotes, horse, ox, goat, etc.). (Psoroptes communis, horse, ox, sheep, etc.). (Sarcoptes equi, canis, suis, cati, etc.). (Sarcoptes mutans of fowl). (Acarus folliculorum or Demodex folliculorum, var. canis, suis, etc.).

[*The common hen louse, Menopon pallidum, is remotely related to the trichodectes, and resembles them in general appearance. It is said to pass readily to other species of birds, and to trouble horses kept near lousy henroosts.]

Fig. 8.

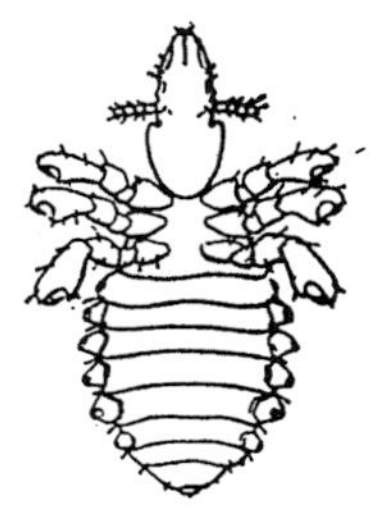

Haematopinus equi.
Blood-sucking Louse.
x 12

Fig. 9.

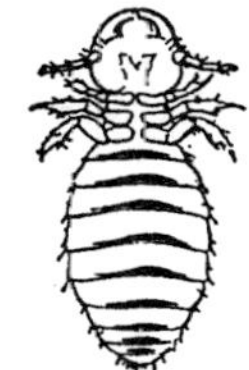

Trichodectes equi.
Scale-eating Louse.
x 20

Fig. 10

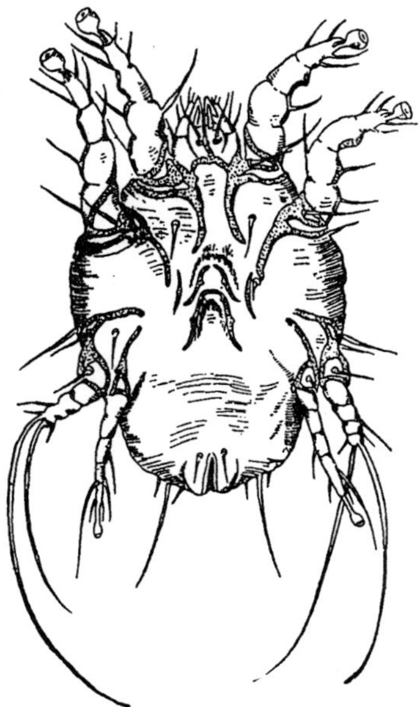

Symbiotes bovis.
Ventral side.
x 100

Fig. 11.

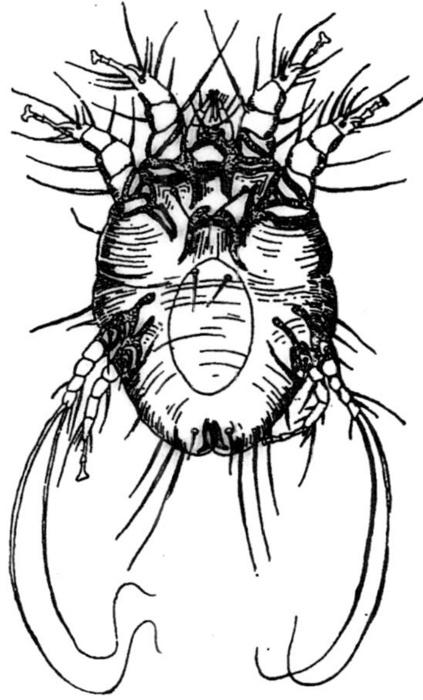

Psoroptes communis.
Ventral surface, Egg in Oviduct.
x 100

Mange (*scabies*) is a contagious dermatitis due to mites. The principal manges are:

a. **Symbiotic mange** (foot mange). Favorite seats: in the horse, hind limbs, in the ox, root of tail. These mites live on the skin, produce loss of hair, desquamation of epithelium, and intense pruritis, causing the animal to stamp and kick continually. The mites are 0.3—0.5 mm long, head broad. The legs, which are long, are provided at their ends with bell-shaped suckers.

b. **Sarcoptic mange of fowls** (Dermatoryctes mutans). It affects the legs, causing "Scaly Feet." The lower, naked portions of the legs become coated with calcarious, smeary or honey-like, scaly, thick deposits. The mites are 0.2—0.5 mm long, legs short, second pair well removed from first. U-shaped chitinous shield behind head.

c. **Psoroptic mange.** Seen in the horse, sheep and ox. Characterized by great desquamation, the appearance of vesicles and papules, the hair or wool agglutinated by crusts of dried exudate; wool becomes tufted, falls out in patches, intense pruritis. The psoroptes is the largest mange mite, 0.4—0.7 mm long; head long, pointed, the three-jointed legs provided with tulip-shaped suckers.

Fig. 12.

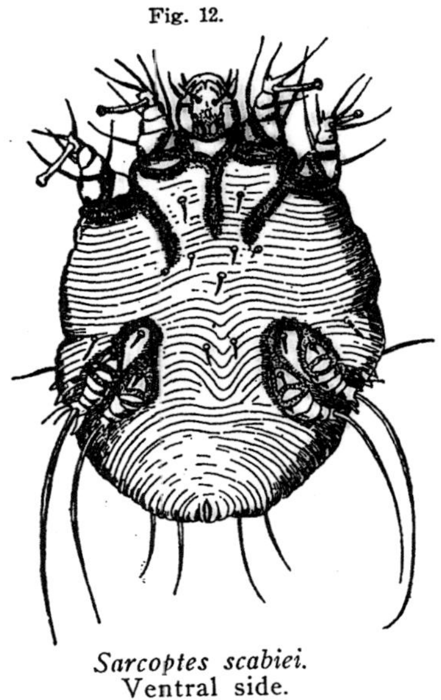

Sarcoptes scabiei.
Ventral side.
x 100

Fig. 13.

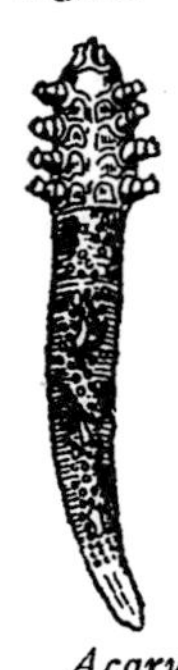

Acarus folliculorum.
x 150

d. **Sarcoptic mange.** Seen in the horse, dog, swine and cat, etc. This mite burrows tunnels in the epidermis, causes nodules, crust formation, thickening and folding of the skin, pruritis. Most difficult mite to capture for microscopical examination; to obtain material for examination the skin should be scraped to bleeding. Sarcoptes are very small, turtle-shaped mites measuring 0.2—0.5 mm head horse-shoe shaped, legs short and stumpy.

e. **Acarus mange.** Most common in dogs and swine, appearing principally on the eyelids, head, extremities, causing little itching. Skin covered with scales, small pustules, and is thickened and folded. In the squamous form circumscribed, bald, bluish-red areas occur, epidermis mother-of-pearl-like, scaly. The parasite is vermiform, 0.2—0.3 mm with a long, narrow, jointed body, the anterior portion carrying four pairs of short, three-jointed feet, at the end of each, three pointed hooks. Eggs spindle-shaped.

III. Skin Diseases Due to Plant Parasites.

Ringworm (Herpes tonsurans) is induced by the fungus Trichopyton tonsurans. The disease is characterized by the appearance of small round, well-defined hairless patches. The smooth skin is covered with grey-colored, asbestos-like crusts. Spontaneous healing begins in the center of the lesion, extending toward the periphery ("ringworm"). Vesicles rarely appear. Most common in the ox. In the crusts and more especially in the hair follicles great numbers of round or ovoid, light-refracting spores can be seen with the aid of the microscope. The spores measure 4u. Some of the spores are arranged in regular order, like a string of beads, others are disposed in irregular groups. The filaments, which may be simple or jointed, show little tendency to branching; their free ends are rounded.

Fig. 14.

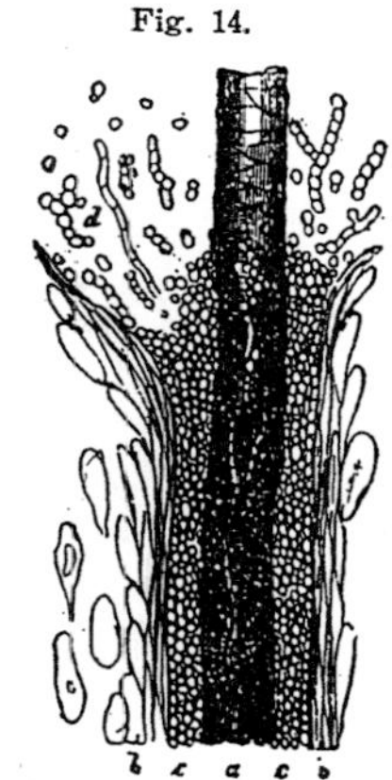

Trichophyton tonsurans.

Favus. Rare, but appears in fowls as so-called "white comb" (Tinea galli). Small whitish-grey spots come upon the comb, which gradually is encrusted by them. In mammals thick, depressed, yellowish brown crusts appear.

Trichorrhexis nodosa is a disease characterized by the formation of nodular enlargements along the shaft of the hair. The hair breaks off at the nodule, leaving a brush-like stump behind. Contagious.

IV. Acute Exanthemas.

1. Foot and mouth disease [said not to occur in the United States], is an acute infectious disease of cloven-hoofed animals, characterized by the appearance of vesicles upon the mucous membrane of the mouth, the skin of the coronet, and in the interdigital space. Period of incubation 1 to 3 days. The disease is attended by moderate fever, salivation, diminished appetite, lameness, recumbent position. The vesicles rupture, leaving erosions

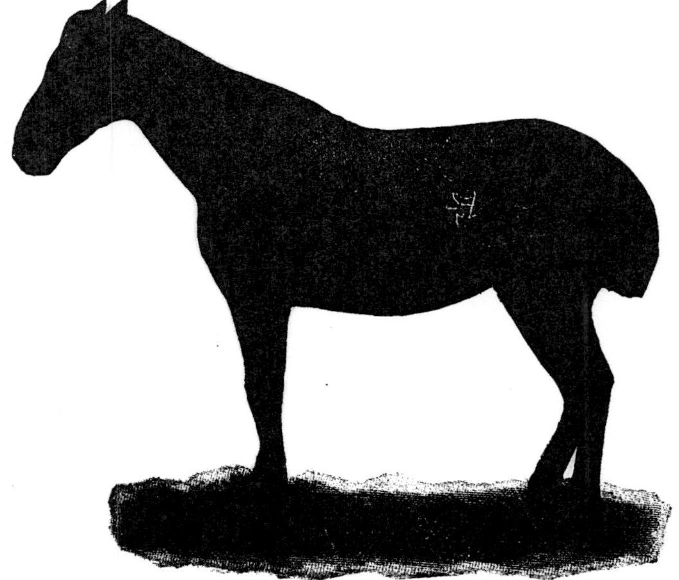

Fig. 15.—Urticaria.

on the mucous membranes, and dry scabs on the skin. Complications are not infrequent.

2. **Sheep pox** is a contagious exanthema running an acute course and having a typical character. Incubation 4 to 7 days; artificial inoculation shorter. On the haired portions of the body, around the eyes, nose, mouth, inner surfaces of the legs, appear punctiform reddenings (pimples), later papules. In about six days the papules are covered by vesicles filled with a clear, tenacious fluid (eruptive stage). In the next few days the contents of the vesicles become turbid, forming pustules (suppurative stage); then drying of the pustules to a solid crust (exsiccative stage). When the crusts fall off a small depressed cicatrix (pit) remains. During the eruption there is fever, loss of appetite, etc. Course about 3 weeks. [Mortality 10 to 50%].

3. **Canadian horse pox.** A contagious pustulous exanthema limited usually to the saddle and harness rests. Period of incubation 2 to 3 days. A few isolated prominences of the size of a half dollar appear, the hair on them is erect and gathered into tufts. The contents of the bullae becomes purulent, erupts, dries to a brownish-yellow solid crust. Caused by a bacillus measuring 2u, which admits of staining with fuchsin.

4. **Urticaria** (nettle rash) is a peracute exanthema which is characterized by its sudden appearance. Tumefactions from the size of a pepper-corn to that of a hand or saucer come upon the neck, head, inner surface of the hind limbs and on the body. They are prominent, flat, soft, warm, the hair upon them standing erect; itching is rare. Urticaria of swine is to be looked upon as a mild form of erysipelas.

5. **Pemphigus acuta.** Noncontagious, benign exanthema characterized by the formation of a limited number of large vesicles (bullae) on different parts of the body.

V. General Diseases which Affect the Skin.

1. **Purpura hemorrhagica** (morbus maculosus) is an acute infectious disease (an intoxication) characterized by the appearance in the various organs of the body, of multiple hemorrhagic centers of varied size. In the absence of complications, the disease is unattended by fever. On the mucous membranes of the nasal passages blood spots are seen, more rarely they occur in the conjunctiva and buccal mucous membranes. In the skin and subcutis of the lips, cheeks, and nostrils, appear hard, inflammatory, edematous swellings from the size of a pigeon's egg to that of a hand (larger by confluence), causing the head of the horse afflicted to

resemble that of a hippopotamus. The extremities also swell, the swellings terminating abruptly at the stifle and the elbow. There is a diffuse edema of the lower abdomen; hemorrhage in the internal organs. Breathing is labored and stentorious from the mechanical obstruction (swelling) to the entrance of air into the upper respiratory passages. There is difficulty in deglutition, colic symptoms, and impaired locomotion. When the disease has existed for several days, the temperature increases. [Course atypical, 6 to 21 days. Mortality about 50%].

VI. Acute Infectious Diseases which Affect the Skin.

1. **Black leg** is an acute infectious disease caused by the entrance of a germ through [the digestive tract or] a lesion in the skin, a peculiar emphysema resulting. On the body, shoulder, neck, upper portions of the extremities (never below the knee or hock) appear swellings which are at first hot and painful, but later cold, painless, emphysematous. Incision causes a foamy, fetid fluid to flow out of them. Attending symptoms are high fever, great depression, lameness, dyspnea. Mortality is high. [Prophylaxis, protective inoculation.]

The bacilli of black leg are contained in the discharges from the swellings. They measure 3—5u long, 0.5—0.6u broad. One end or the middle is enlarged to receive an ovoid spore which it bears. May be stained by Gram's method.

2. **Malignant edema** appears under the same symptoms as black leg; the swellings are more edematous than emphysematous.

The bacillus of malignant edema is somewhat like the bacillus of anthrax, 3.—3.5u long and 1.1u broad. They are mostly united at their ends to form long threads. In the middle of some of the bacilli or at the ends occur spindle or drumstick-like enlargements to receive the ovoid spore. The spore does not accept ordinary stains.

3. **Bovine pest** (Wild- und Rinderseuche) is produced by the bacterium of hemorrhagic septicemia and appears in the exanthematous, pectoral, or intestinal forms. On the head and neck appear large inflammatory edematous swellings, which spread to the mucous membranes of the mouth and throat. The pectoral form is attended by a croupous-hemorrhagic pneumonia with pleuritis, and the intestinal form with hemorrhagic enteritis and swelling of the intestinal viscera. The *Bacterium septicemiae haemorrhagicae*, like that of contagious pneumonia of swine and of chicken cholera, is 0.6u long, 0.3u broad, oval, stains only at the ends, an unstained belt remaining.

4. Examination of the Conjunctiva.

The examination of the conjunctiva serves to determine the quantity and condition of the circulating blood.

Method. Avoid all rough and hasty manipulations. Before grasping the eyelid gain the animal's confidence by arranging the foretop and gently stroking the forehead. The right eyelid should be lifted with the fingers of the left hand, the left one with those of the right hand. By means of the thumb the upper eyelid is raised, the index finger then replaces the thumb, and by gently pressing the everted lid inwardly, the mucous membrane of the upper eyelid and the membrana nictitans become visible. The thumb, which is now free, draws the lower lid downward. The other three fingers may be rested against the zygomatic arch, steadying the hand. (See figure 16).

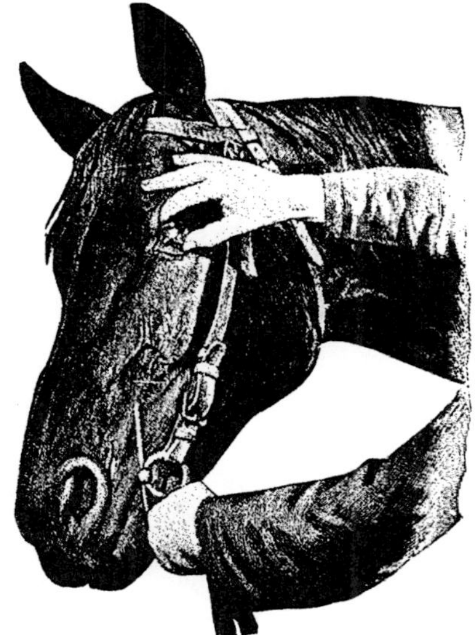

Fig. 16.

In the ox a good view of the scleral conjunctiva may be obtained by simply taking hold of a horn and the nose, and drawing the head to one side.

If we wish to arrive at the condition of the blood from an examination of the mucous membrane of the eye, that organ must be free from local irritation. Severe exercise, and high atmospheric temperature cause a healthy mucous membrane to appear very red from physiological congestion; local inflammation also produces congestions.

A careful comparison of both eyes will enable us to determine the presence of local inflammation. In healthy animals the color of the conjunctiva is pale-roseate; in the ox paler than in other animals. A few blood vessels are always visible. In the conjunctiva, the boundary between normal and diseased conditions is not sharply drawn, hence practice alone makes one capable of giving a reliable judgment.

I. **Discharge from eyelids.** Although mostly due to local diseases, some of the infectious diseases have discharges from the eyelids constantly present. The discharge is either *bilateral* (from both sides) or *unilateral* (from one side only). Bilateral discharges are seen in: malignant head catarrh (with keratitis), Rinderpest (no keratitis present), dog distemper, fowl cholera, influenza. (Swelling shuts off the tear ducts, strangles). Unilateral discharges occur: in continued chronic nasal catarrh, a symptom of glanders, chronic nasal or sinus catarrh. In all animals showing unilateral discharge from the eyelids, especially when the discharge is copious, a careful examination for foreign bodies should be made].

II. **Color.** The color of the conjunctiva is due to the quantity of blood circulating in the blood vessels of the organ and the amount of hemoglobin contained in the blood corpuscles.

1. A *pale, anemic* color shows that the animal is either deficient in blood or that the blood does not contain its normal quota of red corpuscles. The color varies from reddish-white to greyish-white or white.

Paleness occurs *suddenly*:

Following great loss of blood, internal hemorrhages (liver, heart, large blood vessels, etc).

In congestion of blood in the intestines (embolism of intestinal arteries, displacement or torsions of the bowels).

Paleness appears as a *chronic condition*:

In constitutional diseases of the blood-making organs (leucemia, hydremia).

In all chronic diseases which lead to anemia or hydremia, glanders, tuberculosis, distomatosis (liver flukes) and parasitic diseases of the stomach and lungs of sheep.

2. *Venous engorgement* does not always come from plethora. It may *be ramiform, diffuse or punctiform*, and varies in color from a brick red to dark red (cyanotic).

a. *Ramiform congestion* from disease occurs:

In congestion of the head due to hyperemia of the brain, encephalitis. The blood vessels are plainly marked in the diffusely reddened conjunctiva.

When the return of the venous blood from the head is retarded. Characterized by distension of the veins. Occurs in organic heart diseases, heart's weakness, pulmonary emphysema.

b. A diffuse, faded bluish-red discoloration of the conjunctiva is found in conditions leading to an overcharging of the blood with CO_2. It is seen in febrile diseases (infectious diseases), and wherever air is prevented from passing freely into the lungs: diseases of the respiratory tract, respiratory muscles, or heart.

Inflammation of the mucous membrane of the gastro-intestinal tract in the course of colic, produces a cyanotic conjunctiva; if fever appears it becomes ramiform (a bad sign).

c. Spotted or punctiform reddening is almost always due to hemorrhage in the conjunctiva. The color is, therefore, bluish-red and the form round or streaked (petechia, ecchymoses). Seen in purpura hemorrhagica, anthrax, severe anemia and in pernicious anemia.

3. Yellow (*icteric*) discoloration (*jaundice*)

is best observed on the scleral conjunctiva. It is not noticeable by artificial light. If the conjunctiva is pale (bloodless), the yellow can be more readily appreciated. The shades vary from a mere trace of yellow to pronounced lemon yellow; in most cases combined with congestion. The icteric discoloration is due to the abnormal amount of bile coloring matter found free in the blood serum.

According to the origin of the yellow coloring matter we distinguish:

1. *Hematogenous icterus* originates from a dissolution of the red blood corpuscles, the coloring matter becoming set free and mixing with the blood serum. Hematogenous icterus is really a hemoglobinemia. The dissolved blood coloring matter (the methemoglobin) is not changed to bile pigment in the blood, but in the liver. If this organ is able to convert all of the coloring matter to bile and excrete it through the bile ducts, the urine will contain no bile, but the feces will become stained by it (*hypercholia*) and assume a dark color. It may happen, however, that the bile becomes so thick that it congests the smaller bile ducts, is reabsorbed and stains the urine.

Hematogenous icterus is seen in influenza of the horse, azoturia, pyemia, septicemia [Texas fever], and in certain cases of poisoning, especially after prolonged chloroform narcosis.

2. *Hepatogenous icterus* is due to the free flow of bile from the liver becoming retarded (biliary stasis) and its passing over into the blood (cholemia) via lymph vessels and thoracic duct. The obstruction may have its seat in the biliary capillaries or larger ducts, and often at the termination of the *ductus choledochus* in the bowel. Hepatogenous icterus is characterized by the appearance of bile pigments in the urine while the feces, containing less than normal, are of too light a color.

Hepatogenous icterus is seen in duodenal catarrhs with swelling and mucous obstruction of the *ductus choledochus,* tumors, parasites (ascarides) and concretions which block the bile flow. In lupinosis and phosphorous poisoning a swelling of the ducts and parenchyma of the liver occurs leading to the collection and absorption of bile.

Malignant icterus (*icterus gravis*) has associated with it mental depression and slow heart's action due to the effect of the cholic and other acids contained in bile.

III. Swelling. Swellings of the conjunctiva usually are diffuse and may occur in both eyes. They are due to a serous infiltration of the mucosa and submucosa. If of an inflammatory character they are hot and painful. This condition finds its best development in influenza of the horse, the greatly swollen, glassy mucous membrane protruding from between the half-closed lids. It is seen further in contagious pleuropneumonia of the horse, purpura hemorrhagica, malignant head catarrh of the ox, Rinderpest, anthrax, dog distemper, chicken diphtheritis and strangles.

The swelling may be due to hydremia, as in primary anemia and in cachectic diseases of sheep: liver fluke disease, lung and stomach worm plague.

In the course of chronic diseases of the stomach and intestines a slight swelling of the conjunctiva, attended with a washed-muddy and sometimes icteric discoloration, appears.

The conjunctiva may be drier than normal in severe febrile diseases and bad colics.

5. Bodily Temperature.

The internal temperature of the body is maintained, with slight variation, at a definite elevation by means of an especial regulating apparatus. The production of heat in the body and the loss of heat from the body are kept equal. If the temperature varies from the normal, and this variation be preserved for a time, a disturbance due to disease is affecting the regulatory apparatus.

The determination of the internal temperature is of great importance in the diagnosis of disease, for each deviation from the normal is to be considered a symptom of considerable moment. In all diseases affecting internal organs, the measuring the temperature is imperative.

Method of examination. Thermometry. Formerly the temperature was approximated by laying the hand upon different parts of the body, namely the nose, ears, horns, extremities, or by inserting the fingers into the mouth. Such methods require long practice before a reliable estimate can be obtained, and they are always deceptive. Only in exceptional cases are they now in vogue. The temperature is most accurately measured with a thermometer, graduated in degrees and tenths of a degree. [Except in America, England and perhaps one other country the Celsius (centigrade) thermometer is in common use. It is graduated into 100 degrees, and these subdivided into tenths of a degree. In this country the Fahrenheit thermometer is generally used. It is graduated into 212 degrees, each degree being subdivided into fifths. Our preference for this latter instrument is largely traditional, and it is being displaced by the centigrade, which is now almost universally employed in scientific work.

The following simple formula will indicate how readily the Celsius scale may be converted into the Fahrenheit scale and *vice versa*:

$$\text{Celsius} = 5/9\ (F-32).$$
$$\text{Fahrenheit} = 9/5\ C + 32.$$

For veterinary practice a maximum thermometer should be used, preferably a tested or compared instrument. The thermometer should be inserted full length into the rectum, which gives the best results, though in exceptional cases the vagina is chosen.

We should, of course, guard against being kicked by the animal, and exercise care that the instrument does not break and injure the mucous membrane. Before introducing the thermometer, the column of mercury should be shaken down. The use of water, saliva or oil facilitates insertion. We should allow the instrument to remain in the rectum from three to five minutes.

In fowls the thermometer may be inserted in the rectum as in other animals, or placed under the wing.

Taking the bodily temperature once daily is of great value during the course of an internal disease; in important cases the temperature should be registered twice a day (8 A. M. and 5 P. M.). After diagnostic inoculations (tuberculin, mallein), especially during the critical period, the temperature should be recorded at least every two hours. Thermometry is of great diagnostic importance during an outbreak of an infectious disease, the elevation in temperature being often the first symptom shown. By taking the temperature once daily (best at evening), the infected animals may be determined before further symptoms of disease develop; [influenza, contagious pleuropneumonia, swine plague or hog cholera [Texas fever].

I. The Normal Temperature. The normal temperatures of the different animals are as follows:

Horse	..37.5—38.5° C.	[99.5—101.3° F.]
Ox	....38.0—39.5° "	[100.4—103.1° "]
Sheep	..39.0—40.5° "	[102.2—104.9° "]
Goat	...39.0—40.5° "	[102.2—104.9° "]
Hog	...38.0—40.0° "	[100.4—104.0° "]
Dog	...37.5—39.0° "	[99.5—102.2° "]
Fowls	..41.5—42.5° "	[106.7—108.5° "]

The temperature will vary a few tenths of a degree in the same species, and slight variations may occur in one and the same animal within a single day. This latter variation may amount to 1° C. [1.8° F.].

In healthy but pregnant cows the temperature may vary 1.5° C. [2.7° F.]; a temperature elevation, therefore, of 40.5° C. [104° F.] would not necessarily mean fever in these animals.

When the organs (muscles, glands) are active a slight rise in temperature takes place, when at rest a slight sinking follows.

From long continued exercise at a rapid gait the temperature of a horse may rise 2.5° C. [4.5° F.]. Two hours may elapse before it reaches normal again.

High atmospheric temperatures or warm stables, inasmuch as they reduce radiation, tend to increase the temperature. As a rule the temperature is lower in the morning than toward evening.

Age, race, sex, temperament and when eating have but little influence on bodily temperature. During the hot season of the year, in cattle kept in stables the temperature may rise 1.0° C., for a short time.

As a rule the bodily temperature is lowest in the morning and in the afternoon at about five o'clock highest.

II. Temperature of the skin. The thinner and more vascular the integument and the finer the hair coat, the warmer the organ feels. Exposed surfaces of the skin feel cooler than more protected, covered parts. The ears and extremities, therefore, are normally colder than the rest of the body, as is also true of the comb and legs of fowls.

The surface temperature is measured by laying our hands on the patient, namely on the ears, horns, nose, muzzle and legs. Deviations from the normal, especially in cattle, are sometimes more appreciable by this method than by the use of the thermometer.

A changing of the surface temperature of a given part from hot to cold and *vice versa* is characteristic of fever.

The surface temperature is elevated (skin hot) in fever and during normal outbreak of sweat. It is reduced (skin cold) when the temperature is below normal (milk fever), collapse, during chill stage of fever and in the cold sweat which usually precedes death.

III. Fever. Although the character of fever is not expressed entirely by elevation of temperature, we have become accustomed to associate *high temperature* and *fever*, using the terms as if synonymous. As a matter of fact, the increased temperature is only one of the characteristic and most readily available symptoms in the complex phenomenon called fever. As a rule, however, there is a direct relationship existing between the height of the temperature and the degree of development of the fever. At times in the ox, the increase of temperature, as measured by the thermometer, fails to correspond with the degree of fever, which can be appreciated by the remaining symptoms.

Besides mere increase in temperature, the following phenomena attend fever:

1. *Chill.* When the temperature of the body rises very rapidly the peculiar symptoms of chill are shown: pronounced trembling of the muscles, which can shake the whole body, arched back, erect hair coat, cold skin. Chill is not a constant symptom of fever, occurring only in certain infectious diseases, such as anthrax, Rinderpest, septicemia, pyemia, malignant head catarrh. [It is sometimes seen in animals reacting to tuberculin or mallein].

2. *Uneven distribution of the external temperature of the body.* The ears, horns, nose and extremities are abnormally warm or cold, one extreme alternating with the other. The muzzle of the ox, the nose of the dog and the snout of the hog are dry, even creviced and alternately too hot or too cold.

3. *Acceleration of the pulse and respirations* take place more slowly than the increase in temperature; and they do not bear the same relationship to the temperature in all fevers. The higher the pulse frequency, the more serious the fever, the pulse becoming weak and the artery soft.

4. *Loss of appetite* and impaired digestion. In fever the secretion of the digestive juices is lessened, peristalsis suppressed (constipation), thirst increased.

5. *Mental depression.*

6. *Albuminuria.*

Although the variations in the normal temperature of a given animal are confined to narrow limits, when the temperature exceeds these limits we are not always justified in assuming the presence of fever. The physiological functions of the organs can momentarily become sufficiently accelerated to produce a degree of temperature in excess of the usual normal one. The appearance of concomitant symptoms or repeated recording of the temperature will generally decide whether fever be present or not. In doubtful cases we speak of *high normal temperature.*

The following temperatures may be safely assumed to indicate fever:

In the horse a temperature of 39.0° [102.2° F.] and over.
In the ox " 40.0° [104.9° F.] "
In the dog " 39.2° [102.5° F.] "

In the ox and dog fever is often present without a rise of temperature. In such cases we must depend upon the surface temperature and the other symptoms of fever present.

Generally the height of the temperature expresses the

Fig. 17.

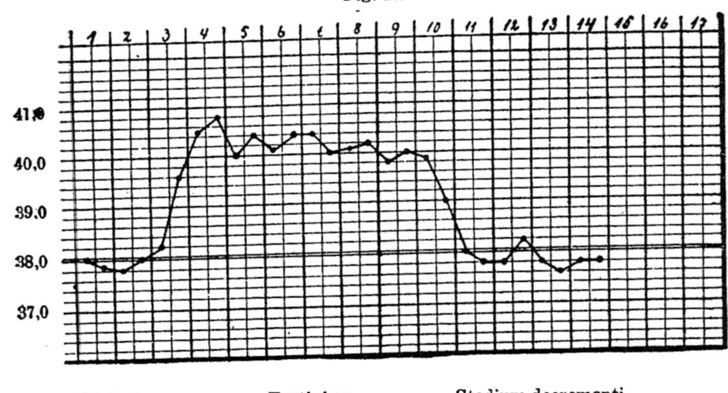

Stad. incre-menti | Fastigium. | Stadium decrementi. Crisis

Febris continua—Equine Pleuro-pneumonia.

height of the fever. Four degrees of fever are distinguished, which for the horse and dog are as follows:

1. *Mild fever* 38.5°—39.5° C. [101.3°—103.1° F.].
2. *Moderate fever* 39.5°—40.5° C. [103.1°—104.9° F.].
3. *High fever* 40.5°—41.5° C. [104.9°—106.7° F.].
4. *Very high fever* or hyperpyretic temperature 41.5° C. [106.7° F.] and over.

Usually in the horse even in the most severe infectious diseases, the temperature does not exceed 41.7° C. [107.0°

F.]; only exceptionally, in tetanus, contagious pleuropneumonia, and influenza, is this high mark passed. The highest temperature is carried by fowls, namely 43,5° C. [110,3° F.]. [In cases of "heat stroke" in horses hyperpyretic temperature may reach 110° F.].

During a single day a febrile temperature does not remain constant, but agreeing with the variations of the normal temperature, is lower in the morning than toward evening—the so-called morning *remissions* and evening *exacerbations.*

Fig. 18.

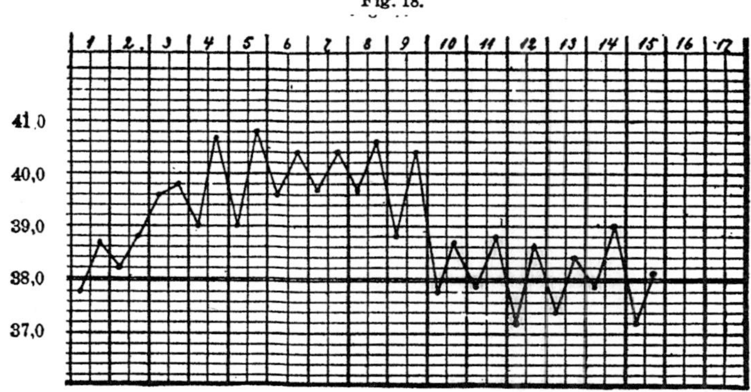

Febris remittens.—South African Horse Sickness.

Recording of the variations in temperature which occur during the course of a disease is also of great importance. If the temperature is measured at a certain time daily and the record expressed in a graphic manner, the so-called fever curve is obtained. From the fever curve is recognized the type of fever present.

In veterinary medicine the following types of fever are important:

1. *Continued* fever, daily variation less than 1° C. (1.8° F.).

2. *Remittent* fever, daily variation over 1° C.

3. *Intermittent* fever, periodical temporary fall to normal temperature.

4. *Atypical* fever is one having no regular character.

Fig. 19.

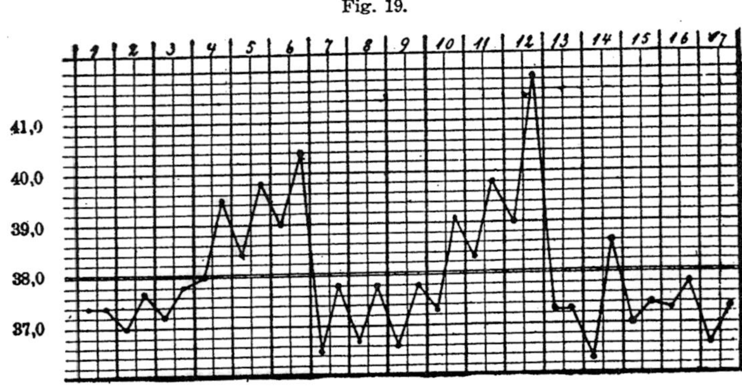

Febris intermittens—Flagelosis of the Horse.

In the course of most infectious diseases, three stages are distinguished, according to the course of the fever, viz.:

Fig. 20.

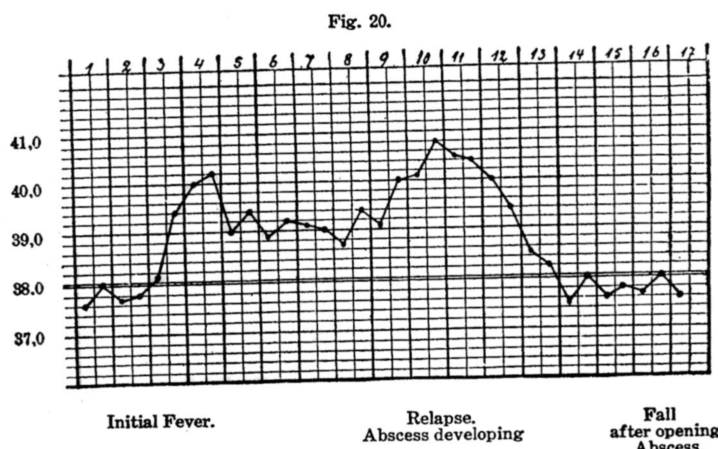

Febris atypica—Strangles of the Horse.

1. *Stage of increasing temperature* (stadium incrementi).

2. *Acme,* temperature at its highest (fastigium).

3. *Stage of falling temperature* (stadium decrementi).

A rapid fall of temperature (within 1-2 days) is called *crisis,* a gradual decline, *lysis.*

According to duration we distinguish: *ephemeral* (one day), *acute* and *chronic* fevers.

IV. Subnormal Temperature. Hypothermia. Like the high normal, the subnormal temperature may be physiological. It may come from the fact that the *sphincter ani* is relaxed, or that the thermometer has not been inserted deep enough, or that the rectum is filled with feces, or that defecation takes place just before or during the insertion of the instrument.

A subnormal temperature due to disease is uncommon. It is seen to occur, but not constantly, in parturient paresis, certain gastro-intentinal diseases of the dog, anemia, hemorrhage, *icterus gravis.* A subnormal temperature is most frequent in fatal diseases just before death (temperature of collapse).

General Infectious Diseases.

Septicemia. Nearly all forms of so-called "Blood Poisonings" are designated by the collective term *Septicemia.* Symptoms: suddenly appearing fever, often accompanied by chill; fever of the continued type; mucous membranes highly reddened, often icteric, frequently ecchymosed. Very rapid, small pulse. Food and drink refused; fetid diarrhea. Great mental depression, blank countenance, eyes sunken. Acute or peracute course.

Pyemia is a general disease due to *pus cocci* gaining access to the blood, and is characterized by multiple, secondary abscess formation (pyemic metastasis) in the various organs, lungs, liver, kidneys, brain, joints, etc. Diagnosis is easy when primary abscess is available; otherwise it is difficult. As each new abscess forms the temperature increases, therefore it is fever of intermittent type. Mucous membranes are congested, icteric. Pulse is continued high. Course subacute.

Anthrax is an acute infectious disease due to the *Bacillus anthracis.* Begins suddenly with high fever; tendency toward hemorrhages from mucous membranes. In the ox and sheep the course is often apoplectic; when course is acute it lasts 1-3 days. Brain symptoms, convulsive twitchings of muscles, rapid pulse, dyspnea, loss of milk, are symptoms sometimes seen. In horse, colic symptoms occur. Formation of anthrax carbuncle in skin is not rare in the horse. In hog, symptoms of severe laryngo-pharyngitis with swelling predominate. Diagnosis is positive only after finding bacilli under the microscope. An anthrax slide is made as follows: A thin layer of blood or spleen pulp is smeared over a slide, passed three times through the flame of a Bunsen burner, then covered with a 2% watery solution of safranin and allowed to boil by holding over a Bunsen flame for a few moments. Wash and examine.

Fig. 21.

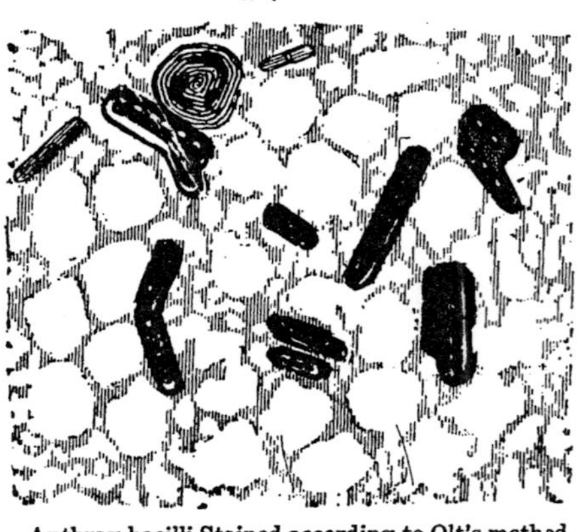

Anthrax bacilli Stained according to Olt's method. a. b., Cadaver bacilli.

The anthrax bacilli are from 1 to 2 times as long as the diameter of a red blood corpuscle, and are composed of from 2 to 8 bacterial cells, which are stained reddish brown on the slide. Each bacterial cell is cylindrical, slightly longer than broad, appearing almost square in form. The ends are plane or somewhat convex. The bacterial cells are surrounded by a gelatinous capsule, which is stained yellow in the preparation, and which joins the cells together to form the bacillus. The capsule is bounded by a dark line. If the bacilli come in contact with one another they unite, their capsules blending together.

Influenza. An acute, infectious disease of the horse, very easily transmitted. Period of incubation 5 to 7 days. First symptom is a rise in temperature which continues 3 to 6 days, then crisis. Great debility, slow gait, staggering, great mental depression, head held down or rested on manger, eyelids and conjunctiva swollen, hot, painful, photophobia. Pulse at first strong, little affected, later accelerated. Loss of appetite, diarrhea in about 3 days. In later stages cold, painless edematous swelling of the extremities. Mortality 4%.

[**Hog Cholera.** Infectious disease of swine, caused by bacilli which enter the body through the respiratory tract, or via respiratory tract or mouth—

with food and water—(hog cholera of Smith). Period of incubation 4 to 21 days. Young pigs most predisposed. One attack produces immunity in most cases. Symptoms: apoplectic form; die very suddenly or after a few hours illness (beginning of an outbreak). Usual form: fever, temperature 107°-108°F., appetite impaired, tremblings of muscles, unwillingness to move, stupid, dull, hide in litter. Bowels at first constipated; later diarrhea. Eyelids filled with mucus. Respiration accelerated, labored; painful, frequent cough. On pendant parts of body, skin is reddened, congested; eczematous eruptions, ulceration of skin. Rapid loss of flesh, unsteady, tottering gait. Death within 48 hours to 2 weeks. Mortality 20-100%.

Texas Fever. An infectious blood disease of the ox caused by a protozoön (*Pyrosoma bigeminum*) which enters and destroys the red blood corpuscles. The disease is spread by the cattle tick, *Boöphilus bovis,* the younger generation of which carries the protozoön. Period of incubation 13-90 days **after exposure to tick-infected places.** Symptoms: fever (104°-109° F), unnatural recumbent positions and standing attitudes; animal is dull, stupid; in some cases shows vicious tendencies; horns, ears, and hoofs are hot. Pulse is rapid; dyspnea; constipation, excreta tinged with bile. Visible mucous membranes icteric. In later stages urine red. Ticks of various size to be found on escutcheon, inside of thighs, base of udder or scrotum. Little blood flows from intentional wounds. Characteristic post-mortem changes. Duration 3 days to several weeks. Mortality 20-90%].

Chicken cholera. Attacks all kinds of fowls. Incubation period one day. Birds sit languidly on the ground, feathers ruffled, eyelids closed and stuck with exudate. Temperature 42-43.2° C. Respirations increased, jerky, and often noisy. Appetite lost. Thirst increased. Feces watery, greenish, yellow or bloody, mixed with mucus and fetid. Death in three days with sinking temperature. Often apoplectic death.

Chicken pest is an acute, very transmissible infectious disease, generally distributed. Affects usually only chickens and clinically and pathologically very like cholera. The patients never show diarrhea, the course is slower and apoplectic death does not occur. The virus, contrary to chicken cholera, is ultramicroscopic.

Hemorrhagic septicemia (Wild-und Rinderseuche) is an acute, general infectious disease appearing in the exanthematous, pectoral and intestinal form. High fever. In cattle a hard, inflammatory-hemorrhagic edema of the head and swelling of the tongue occurs. Dyspnea.

Swine erysipelas (Rotlauf) is an acute, infectious disease, usually fatal. Incubation period 3-5 days. Sudden fever, great languor, weakness of the hind parts, stupor. Patients burrow in straw. Vomiting. Skin between thighs, under belly, neck and chest diffusely reddened. Dyspnea. Death in four days.

Braxy of Sheep. A peracute hemorrhagic inflammation of the abomasum due to the **bacillus gastromycosis ovis.** In many respects resembles anthrax.

South African Horse Sickness. A non-contagious (though readily transmittable by blood inoculation) disease of horses and mules. Incubation 7 days. Slowly rising fever with morning remissions. Symptoms of pulmonary edema (Dumperre zickte) or swelling of the head (Dikkop). Great muscular weakness, animals recumbent. Pulse not very rapid but small. Mortality 80-90%.

B. The Special Part of the Examination.

6. Circulatory Apparatus.

An examination of the circulatory apparatus is of importance not only to diagnose those maladies which affect the organs carrying the blood, but also from the fact that *all acute* general or infectious diseases of a serious character influence more or less greatly the circulation.

A methodical examination of the organs carrying the blood includes:

I. Taking the pulse.

II. Noting the condition of the peripheral blood vessels.

III. Examining the heart.

I. Pulse.

Method of Examination. The pulse is felt with the fingers, which may be gently rested upon any of the superficial arteries having bone or other hard tissue under them. In the horse and ox the sub-maxillary artery is most commonly used, in the latter animal the artery is easily felt on the lateral side of the jaw bone. Other arteries which may be used to take the pulse are the radial, plantar, temporal, transverse facial and coccygeal. In the dog, sheep, goat and cat the femoral artery is most available. [In dogs and cats the brachial artery can be felt on the medial surface of the humerus, just in front of and above the elbow.] In the hog and fowl the pulse can not be felt, hence the heart's beat is used.

To palpate the pulse place the first, second and third fingers over the artery, pressing it slightly and rolling it somewhat under the fingers. Before one can judge the pulse, several beats must be felt, best counting them for a full minute.

From a clinical standpoint the 1. *Frequency,* 2. *Rhythm,* and 3. *Quality,* are of importance to consider in examining the pulse.

a. *Frequency*. By the frequency of the pulse we mean the number of blood-waves (beats) felt in a minute's time. There is a great variation in the normal frequency, not only in the different species of animals, but also in animals of the same kind. Many physiological conditions have great influence upon the pulse-frequency: size, age, sex, race, atmospheric temperature, time of day, prehension or digestion of food, exercise, excitement, are all factors.

Large animals carry a slower (less frequent) pulse than small ones; adults slower than young; females higher (more frequent) than males; well bred individuals, slower than mongrels; in summer the pulse is higher than in winter; in the morning slower than toward evening; excited animals show a more rapid pulse than animals standing at perfect rest. In nervous animals (horses and dogs) the act of taking the pulse often increases its frequency.

Taking these physiological variations into consideration, the following is the average pulse-frequency for the different animals.

1.	Horses in general	28— 40.
	Warm blooded stallions	28— 32.
	Cold blooded stallions	28— 36.
	Colts, two weeks old	—100.
	" four weeks old	— 70.
	" six to twelve months old	45— 60.
	" two to three years old	40— 50.
2.	Asses and mules	45— 50.
3.	Bovines	40— 80.
4.	Sheep and goats	70— 90.
*5.	Swine	60—100.
6.	Dogs	60—120.
7.	Cats	110—130.
*8.	Fowls	120—160.

*NOTE. The numbers refer to the heart's beat, as the pulse can not be felt in swine and fowls.

In regard to frequency we distinguish a slow pulse (*pulsus rarus*) and a rapid pulse (*pulsus frequens*).

The slow pulse (*pulsus rarus, bradycardia*) is very uncommon. It most often accompanies brain diseases attended by great depression (chronic and subacute hydrocephalus, tumors in the brain), icterus gravis, and poisoning from alcohol or lead. In the horse at times it is seen in gastro-intestinal affections with loss of appetite, probably due to some alteration in the sympathetic nerve.

Fig. 22.

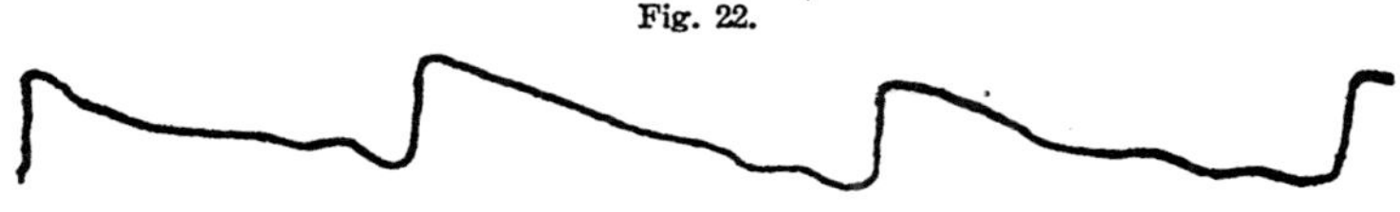

Slow, Sluggish Pulse of Horse.
Taken with Marey's Sphygmograph--Art transversa faciei.

The fast pulse (*pulsus frequens, tachycardia,*) is very common in disease. A very rapid pulse, though characteristic of no special disease, is always *a sign that the parenchyma of the heart is affected,* hence in severe diseases it is an index to the heart's strength. Rarely in the horse does the pulse frequency exceed 80 beats per minute; if it exceed 100, the prognosis is unfavorable. In the ox a pulse of 100, and in the dog one of 120-150 denotes severe illness.

An abnormally accelerated pulse occurs:

1. In all severe diseases, especially when attended by fever. The frequency of the pulse, however, does not always bear the same relationship to the height of the temperature; whether the pulse be accelerated or not depends upon the fever's effect upon the heart, which differs with the disease present. In contagious pleuropneumonia of the horse, septicemia, anthrax, and severe inflammations of the bowels and peritoneum, the pulse rate corresponds to the height of the fever; in influenza and in strangles, the acceleration of pulse is not marked, compared with the temperature.

2. In painful conditions (severe injuries, fractures of bones, abscess in hoof, etc.).

3. In mental excitement (fear, anxiety).

4. In severe hemorrhage.

b. *Rhythm.* When the individual pulse beats are separated by intervals of equal duration, the pulse is regular (*pulsus regularis*). In the dog and, according to Cadeac, frequently in mules and asses, the pulse is often irregular and intermittent.

Fig. 23.

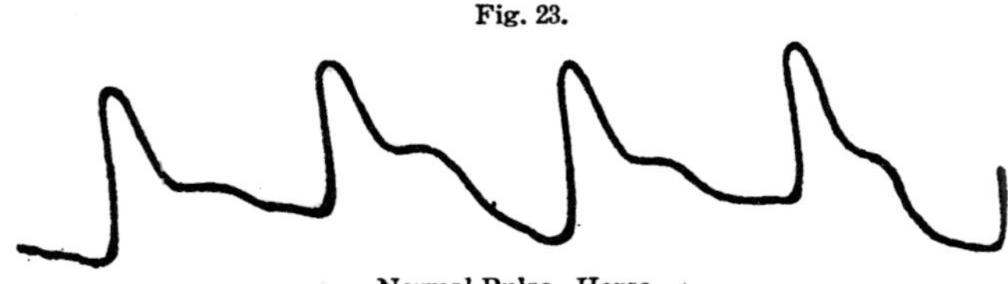

Normal Pulse—Horse.
Marey's Sphygmograph—Art. trans. faciei.

The rhythm of the irregular and of the intermittent pulse is abnormal, i. e., *arhythmic.*

When the pulse is irregular the intervals between the individual pulse beats are of unequal duration.

This is due to lack of innervation of the heart, as well as to exhaustion of the organ. If the pulse of the horse exceeds 80 it is usually irregular. Irregularity is also observed in valvular diseases of the heart, and in myocarditis.

The pulse is *intermittent* when a beat fails now and then. When *regularly intermittent,* a certain beat can not be felt, as for instance, every fourth or fifth pulse wave; when *irregularly intermittent* there is a lapse which does not occur between any certain beats.

The intermittent pulse is commonly physiological, and seen in perfectly healthy horses and dogs, where it disappears after exercise and, therefore, probably due to lacking innervation. Pathologically it appears in chronic hydrocephalus (dummies), severe gastric troubles, and during convalescence from infectious diseases which have occasioned high pulse (contagious pleuropneumonia of the horse).

c. *Quality.* The pulse beats should be of equal volume. When this is true we speak of an equal pulse (*pulsus aequalis*).

The quality of the pulse varies with the kind of animal. The normal size, strength and hardness of the pulse can only be learned by experience; it can not be defined. In the horse the pulse is large, strong and the artery only moderately tense; in the ox the pulse is smaller, not so strong but the artery is tenser and may be rolled under your finger like a hard rubber tube. In small animals the pulse is quick, strong and hard. (See 76 .) In dogs often it is inequal.

The normal quality of the pulse can suffer change in various ways.

1. According to whether a greater or smaller quantity of blood is forced into the arterial system, we distinguish a full (*pulsus magnus*) and an empty (*pulsus parvus*).

The pulse becomes empty when much accelerated and in severe hemorrhages. In fatal diseases the pulse finally becomes imperceptible (*pulsus insensibilis*), indicating cardiac weakness or anemia.

Fig. 24.

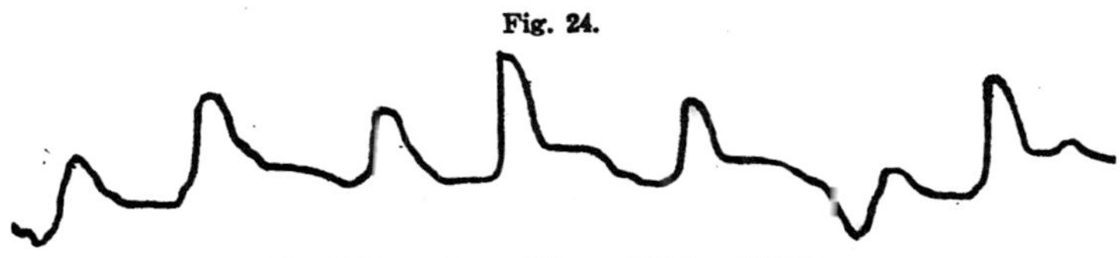

Small, Irregular and Inequal Pulse of Horse.
Marey's Sphygmograph.

2. If the pulse waves are not of equal volume the pulse is called inequal (*pulsus inaequalis*). This is a very important symptom of cardiac weakness, where it is uniformly associated with irregularity, and of valvular (*mitral*) heart

disease. At times there exists a close relationship between an irregular and an inequal pulse. A small wave follows closely a larger one, so that there is a regular alternation of weak and strong beats. It denotes beginning heart's weakness.

3. By the strength of the pulse we mean the force with which it lifts the finger palpating it. We distinguish a strong (*pulsus fortis*) and a weak (*pulsus debilis*). In hypertrophy of the heart the pulse is strong; in parenchymatous degeneration of the cardiac muscle, it is weak. The degree of weakness shown by the pulse indicates the severity of the attack. We form an estimate of the strength of the pulse by noting whether it is readily compressible or not.

4. The hardness of the pulse is due to the distention of the arterial wall and is greatest at the acme of a wave. The pulse is hard (*pulsus durus*) in severe pain, peritonitis, tetanus and acute brain diseases. [In inflammation of serous membranes generally the pulse is hard]. The opposite of a hard pulse is the soft pulse (*pulsus mollis*).

5. As combinations of varied degrees of size, strength and hardness of the pulse are noted, special but superfluous kinds are spoken of: Trembling pulse (*p. tremulus*), where the wave in the distended artery is so small that only a slight trembling can be felt. Thready pulse (*p. filiformis*) is one which is so small, weak and soft as to be hardly perceptible. If associated with this pulse the visible mucous membranes are cyanotic, it shows deficient heart's strength and justifies a bad prognosis. The *wiry* pulse is a small, tense and very hard pulse. Occurring in colic it is a bad sign. A less marked wiry pulse may be noted in aortic stenosis and in chronic nephritis.

6. The arch of the pulse wave may become changed in disease. If the wave is very abrupt, we speak of a hopping, swift pulse (*p. celer*); if, on the contrary, the wave is much prolonged, it is spoken of as a "sluggish" pulse (*p. tardus*).

A quick pulse (*p. celer*) is associated with mild cases of cardiac hypertrophy, plainly marked in aortic insufficiency. In the latter case it is due to the regurgitation of the blood, which occurs at systole, into the hypertrophic left ventricle. In both these instances the pulse is full and strong. Remarkably in heart's weakness a *p. celer* is often present. However, here the pulse is weak and the artery empty. The "sluggish" pulse (*p. tardus*) is noted in very lymphatic horses and is characteristic only of aortic stenosis, when it is at the same time small.

7. A peculiar pulse is the *dicrotic* pulse where two expansions can be felt in one beat of the artery. It is seen in cases of lowered arterial tension combined with weakened heart's action, and is, therefore, noted in long continued fevers and in all forms of anemia.

Fig. 25.

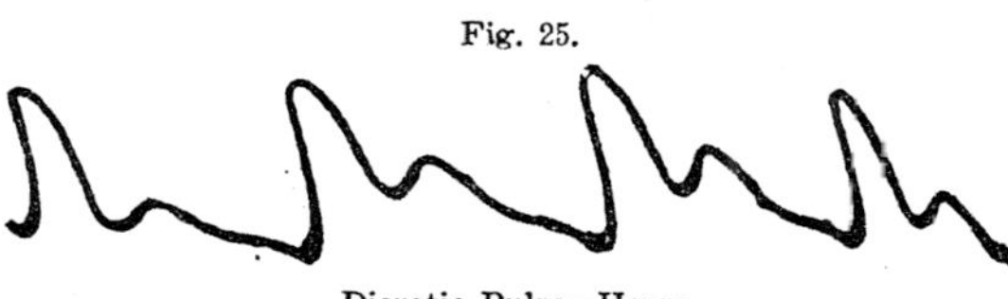

Dicrotic Pulse—Horse.
Marey's Sphygmograph.

II. Examination of the Peripheral Blood Vessels.

Arteries. A strong pulse attending wasting disease and emaciation calls for an examination of the small superficial arteries. An abnormally strong *pulsation in the peripheral arteries of small caliber* is visible in the horse in the branchings of the external maxillary artery.

It appears in hypertrophy of the left ventricle especially when the aortal valves are defective.

Veins. The state of distention of the veins is of primary interest. The veins become prominent after any acceleration of the heart's action in thin-skinned, fine-haired horses; the condition, which is physiological, being a temporary one. *A permanent distention of the veins* is pathological, and is due to an obstruction of the free flow of blood to the right heart. It is mostly plainly visible in the jugulars and their plexus on the head, other superficial veins (external thoracics, milk veins, veins of the extremities) showing it less on account of the edema usually accompanying the condition.

The jugulars can be distended to the size of the human wrist, or even the arm, appearing as great, round strands. The veins of the conjunctiva can also be distended, being recognized as ramiform, often contorted, bluish strands in the mucous membrane.

The veins are generally distended:

1. In valvular disease (tricuspid). It is usually secondary but in the ox mostly primary.

2. In chronic pulmonary diseases interfering with circulation: emphysema.

3. In diseases of the heart's muscle, the organ having become so weak that it is unable to handle the quantity of blood: traumatic myocarditis of the ox.

4. From excessive intrathoracic pressure upon the heart and large blood vessels: tympanitis, pleuritis, pericarditis traumatica of the ox, tumors.

Pulsation in veins. Besides being distended, veins can show pulsation under some circumstances. Synchronous with the respirations, and independent of the heart's action, a slight swelling of the jugulars occurs during the act of expiration, to fall again at inspiration. A so-called *jugular pulse* is normal in the ox for the following reasons: The jugulars and anterior vena cava in this animal are comparatively large. The continual flow of the venous blood into the right heart suffers during the systole of the right auricle, which slightly precedes that of the ventricle, a momentary interruption, the blood congesting in the anterior vena cava and jugulars, causing a brief distention of the jugulars, simulating a pulsation. It is therefore not an active pulsation, but merely a passive undulation due to a regurgitation of the blood in the form of waves. The presystolic appearance of the pulse movement characterizes it, therefore it should always be compared with the arterial pulse. The collapse of the vein is synchronous with the arterial pulse.

The undulation of the jugular vein is intensified in the ox and becomes apparent in other animals when the above cited condition prevails, induced by a morbid congestion of the blood at the heart. In the horse the venous pulse is seen near the aperture of the thorax (lower portion of the neck).

A true (positive) venous pulse is pathological. It is coincident with the heart's systole, and is produced by a defective closing of the atrio-ventricular valves, the blood regurgitating into the auricle. True venous pulse is a characteristic symptom of tricuspid insufficiency.

Fig. 26.

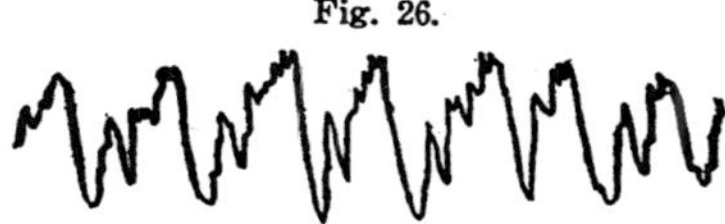

Venous Pulse—Horse.

The valves in the jugulars do not prevent the flowing back of the blood, as they are commonly not well developed, and if the vein be greatly distended they cannot close the lumen of the vessel.

III. The Heart.

The heart is examined by palpation, percussion and auscultation.

Anatomical. In all domestic animals the heart lies in the ventral portion of the thoracic cavity from the third and sixth ribs, in the dog extending to the seventh rib. The great mass of the organ (3-5) lies to the left of the median line, so that it approaches nearer the left thoracic wall than the right one. It does not occupy a perpendicular position, but an oblique one directed from the right, in front and above to the left, backward and downward, the left side of the apex reaching the chest wall.

Horse. The base of the heart lies below the upper half of the height of the chest cavity, resting against the thoracic wall between the 4th and 5th intercostal space. The point of contact occupies a surface of about 10 cm high and 6-8 cm broad. (See Fig. 27, page 87).

Ox and small ruminants. The heart is smaller and does not extend quite as far back as the 6th rib, its base, however, extends to the median line of the chest. Between the 4th and 5th ribs it comes in immediate contact with the thoracic wall. (See Fig. 26.)

Dog. The heart is of rounder form and lies at an angle of 40-45° with the sternum, touching the chest wall along a narrow strip from the 4th to the 7th ribs. The apex is below the 6th intercostal space. (See Fig. —.)

Palpation of the heart's region. The beat of the heart can be felt by laying the flat of the hand over the cardiac region. Inasmuch as the anconeus muscles partly cover the region, the hand should be placed between them and the chest wall. In the depths a dull thud will be felt, produced by the thumping of the heart against the chest wall. The beat is due to a contraction of the heart's muscles which causes a slight torsion of the organ to the left, bringing the left side, not the apex, in contact with the wall of the chest. The beat can best be felt in all animals at the 5th intercostal space, just above the union of the ribs with their cartilages. The force with which the beat can be felt depends upon the condition of the animal as to flesh, it being more plainly marked in thin animals, and just after severe exercise or excitement. Only in the dog can the heart's beat be felt normally on the right side.

In swine and fowls the heart is palpated to determine its action, as the pulse in these animals can not be felt. In swine the heart beats 60-100, and in fowls 120-160 times per minute. Great variations are, however, noted due to the excitability of these animals.

The force of the heart's beat can be increased or diminished. When the force of the beat is much increased a *palpitation* of the heart is spoken of. It occurs:

1. In hypertrophy of the heart (here combined with strong pulse).

2. In heart's weakness, the muscles of the organ undergoing spasm-like contractions incapable of properly propelling the blood to the periphery, the pulse being small. The condition is seen in acute myocarditis, endocarditis and pericarditis.

3. Where the lung between the heart and the chest wall becomes thickened.

The heart's beat is weakened:

1. When the force is enfeebled from degeneration of the heart's muscle.

2. Where the heart is crowded away from the chest wall by accumulations of exudate in the thoracic cavity (pleuritis, pericarditis), or in some cases of pulmonary emphysema or tumors.

Percussion of the heart. Except in very thin animals (horses) the percussion of the heart is of no great value in the diagnosis of disease, the reason being that with the percussion hammer we are unable to determine the boundaries of the organ, the adjacent lung tissues so modifying the sound that the merging of the **dull** sound of the heart's percussion into the **full** sound of the lung's is a very gradual one.

Horse. In the horse, under favorable circumstances, in the region of the 4th and 5th intercostal space a zone of dullness about the size of a hand can be brought out by percussion. Its boundaries, however, are generally indefinite.

Ox. Although the chest walls are thinner in this animal, the heart is covered more by the lungs than in the horse.

Sheep and Goats. A slight dullness is noted over the fifth rib.

Dog. A narrow horizontal line of dullness between the 4th and 7th ribs can be determined on both sides by vigorous percussion.

Due to unfavorable anatomical position, the percussion of the heart is of diagnostic service only in a few instances.

The zone of cardiac dullness is increased in hypertrophy of the heart and where fluids collect in the pericardium; tumors and thickenings of the lungs also induce it.

The zone of cardiac dullness is sometimes decreased from pulmonary emphysema because the distended lung extends further over the heart.

A tympanitic tone on percussion over the cardiac region is obtained in traumatic pericarditis of the ox, gases of putrefaction accumulating in the pericardium.

The percussion of the cardiac region causes the animal pain in pleuritis and pericarditis.

The Auscultation of the Heart.

Method. The auscultation of the heart may be practiced by placing the right ear just behind the left elbow, the leg being drawn forward. Small animals may be laid upon the table and the stethoscope used.

Physiology. In the cardiac region and in the neighborhood of the same, we hear at each action of the heart two tones. One of these tones appears at the moment the organ contracts **(systole)**, and the second tone, which quickly follows the first, at the dilation of the organ **(diastole)**. The second tone follows so closely the first one that it is difficult to differentiate between them, except in animals which carry a pulse below 60. In animals which have a rapid pulse it may be necessary to compare the pulse at a peripheral artery with the heart's beat.

The origin of the heart-tones is still subject to dispute, the authorities not agreeing.

[The first heart-sound (the systolic) is caused by the contracting muscles of the organ and the closing of the auriculo-ventricular valves. The second sound is produced by the closing of the semilunar valves].

The first sound in our domestic animals is duller, deeper, more prolonged and usually louder than the second one, which is short, not so deep, well defined (sharper), not so loud, and at times slightly metallic. There is a great variation in the sound produced by the heart in the different animals, and even in animals of the same species, the sounds being in one case sharper (more metallic) and in another deeper and duller. The thickness of the chest walls is also of influence, in animals with well muscled chests the sounds are seemingly more muffled, duller. By pronouncing the syllables *lub-dub* one can mimic the sounds of the heart.

I II I II

lub dub lub dub

Change in Heart-Sounds Due to Disease.

Both sounds are increased in:

1. Hypertrophy of the heart, the valves remaining intact. (idiopathic hypertrophy).
2. Anemias.

3. A thickening of the lung tissue around the heart, producing a better conductor of sound.

The second sound only is increased:

When the arteries are greatly distended, not infrequently the result of a congestion of the pulmonary circulation combined with hypertrophy of the heart.

Both sounds are weakened when the normal heart becomes enfeebled through disease of its parenchyma, or where the hypertrophic organ is exhausted.

Metallic tones occurring during systole are very common in anemic animals. In traumatic pericarditis of the ox, the pericardium containing gas, a loud metallic tone is heard at each systole when the heart-muscle is still vigorous. Sometimes the sound can be plainly heard the distance of several paces from the affected animal.

This is due to the accumulation of gas in the pericardium acting as a resonant mechanism which augments the sound.

The first tone is *dull* in heart's weakness and in myocarditis, especially noticeable in acute infectious diseases.

A *splitting* |⌣⌣⌣|—⌣⌣| or *doubling* |⌣⌣⌣|—⌣⌣| of the heart sounds, the condition of the circulatory apparatus being otherwise normal, is of no significance. Commonly the first sound is preceded by a short tone ⌣|——⌣|, which is produced by the contracting of an unusually well developed auricle.

Heart bruits. Heart bruits are abnormal sounds and are therefore pathological. They are caused by the sound producing parts of the organ vibrating for too long a time. Endocardial bruits and pericardial bruits are distinguished.

1. Endocardial bruits (noises) come from within the heart and are closely connected with the heart sounds. We can distinguish, therefore, *systolic bruits* and *diastolic bruits,* depending upon whether they occur at the first or second sound. If the bruits are produced by anatomi-

cal changes of the heart itself, they are called *organic,* otherwise *inorganic.*

a. The *organic* or *endocardial* heart bruits are caused either by a narrowing (stenosis) of the atrio-ventricular or arterial openings or by alterations on the valves preventing them from closing properly (insufficiency). They form most valuable symptoms in the diagnosis of heart diseases.

In stenosis the bruit occurs at the moment the blood passes the contracted orifice, the walls of which are set in vibration. If the stenosis involves the atrio-ventricular opening the bruit occurs at diastole, if in the arterial openings, at systole.

In insufficiency the bruit occurs at the moment at which the valves should close. In consequence of their inability to close a regurgitation of the blood takes place, which produces a renewed vibration of the valves, and gives a bruit. If the insufficiency involves the atrio-ventricular valves, the bruit occurs at systole; if the semilunar valves are insufficient the bruit appears at diastole.

The *character of the bruits* is varied, they can be *buzzing, blowing, purring, hissing, humming, sawing, rattling, long* or *short* tones. Insufficiency bruits are generally softer than those due to stenosis. Heart bruits are made more pronounced by an acceleration of the heart's action, therefore the patient should be exercised before examination.

Gmelin recommends **digitalinum verum** subcutaneously to bring out more distinctly heart sounds or casual bruits. The dose for the horse and ox is 0.025—0.05; for the dog 0.002 —0.009. The digitalin is first dissolved in 5ccm of 50% alcohol and then diluted with 20ccm of water.

Systolic bruits |∿∿∿‿| are characteristic of:
- Insufficiency of an atrioventricular valve.
- Stenosis of an arterial opening.

Diastolic bruits |—∿∿| are characteristic of:
- Stenosis of an atrioventricular opening.
- Insufficiency of a semilunar valve.

Although the bruits originate in different parts of the heart, the exact point of origin cannot be determined by auscultation. In the horse and dog valvular lesions have their seat most commonly in the left heart, rarely are they primary in the right heart. In the ox valvular diseases of the right heart are more frequent than of the left one. The atrioventricular valves are more commonly diseased than the semilunar.

b. Contrary to the endocardial, organic bruits, the *inorganic* or *anemic bruits* occur without that any discernible anatomical alteration appears at the orifices or valves of the heart. Inorganic bruits are systolic, soft, blowing and not constant (*accidental*). They tend to disappear and reappear again. Their origin is not well understood. They are nearly always noted in anemic animals.

It is very important to distinguish between organic and inorganic heart bruits, but in practice this is often very difficult. As a rule, soft, systolic bruits (they do not occur during diastole) should be very carefully estimated. Organic heart bruits are always accompanied by hypertrophy and often alteration of pulse, further by a congestion (stasis) in the pulmonary veins and accordingly an increased pressure in the pulmonary artery, whereby the second heart's sound is loud and clapping.

Fig. 27.

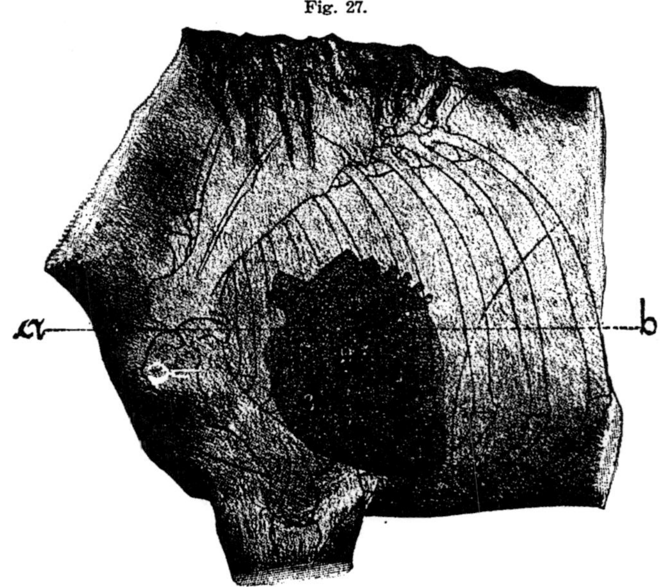

Points at which Endocardial Bruits are most pronounced.
a. b.—Line of Shoulder. 1.—Left Auriculoventricular Opening. 2.—Portal. 3.—Pulmonary Artery.

2. The pericardial bruits. These bruits do not come from within the heart itself, but are extra-cardial. They consist in *frictional* noises due to the pericardium having become so altered that its surface is no longer smooth and slippery, but rough and dry. The bruits are characterized by being *scratching, grating* or *rubbing,* frictional tones not in-

timately related to either systole or diastole. Pericardial bruits, when present, muffle the regular heart sounds.

A pericardial *metallic gurgling* or *liquid* bruit, synchronous with the heart's beat, occurs in the course of traumatic pericarditis when fluid exudate and gas commingle in the pericardium.

Diseases of the Circulatory Apparatus.

Palpitation of the heart (*palpitatio cordis*) is a nervous, transient, greatly increased heart's action not due to any anatomical lesion in the organ. The loud thumping of the heart may shake the thorax and be heard a distance from the body.

Acute myocarditis. A diffuse parenchymatous affection of the heart's muscle which attends severe infectious diseases. Symptoms: great weakness and debility, mucous membranes cyanotic, high fever, heart's beat weak, systolic sound muffled. Pulse very rapid up to 120 in the horse; small, weak arhythmic, inequal, finally imperceptible. Course acute or peracute. Mortality high.

Hypertrophy and dilatation of the heart. Can be present for years without visible symptoms occurring. Symptoms: Pulse strong, also heart impulse, zone of cardiac dullness enlarged on percussion. Later when the heart is greatly dilated and the valves can no longer close sufficiently, symptoms of bicuspid insufficiency occur; pulse rapid, arhythmic, inequal; heart's beat sometimes palpitating, increased dullness on percussion. Systolic blowing bruit, diastolic sound intact or louder than normal. Exercise causes dyspnea from pulmonary venous congestion. Termination as in chronic valvular disease. Most common heart disease of horse and dog.

Acute endocarditis. Not very common. Fever, greatly accelerated heart's action, irregular pulse, intermittent, very small. Heart sounds are at first normal, later systolic bruit. Dyspnea. General condition altered. Prognosis unfavorable.

Valvular disease, chronic endocarditis. Caused by a chronic valvular endocarditis which leads to an atrophy of the valves (insufficiency) or to a narrowing of the orifices (stenosis). Following valvular failure a hypertrophy of the ventricle always takes place; in disease of the semilunar valves the left ventricle, in defects of the mitral valve a hypertrophy of the right ventricle. The hypertrophy of the ventricle, which is combined with dilatation, is compensatory.

B i c u s p i d (Mitral) i n s u f f i c i e n c y. Most common form of heart disease in dogs and horses. Pulse small, irregular. Systolic bruit. Diastolic sound clear, loud. Dyspnea on exercise.

Stenosis of the bicuspid (Mitral) valves. Rare when unattended with insufficiency; an uncommon lesion compared with insufficiency. Pulse small and very weak. Diastolic and pre-systolic bruits. Great dyspnea.

Insufficiency of the tricuspid valves. Rarely primary in the horse, mostly secondary to diseases involving the left ventricle, leading to hypertrophy of the right heart. In the ox frequently primary. Systolic bruits, venous congestion, venous pulse.

Stenosis of the tricuspid valves. Happens only in the ox and is then combined with insufficiency. Diastolic bruits, great venous congestion, dyspnea.

Insufficiency of the aortic semilunar valves. Full, strong, hopping pulse, pulsation in peripheral arteries. Diastolic bruit. Hypertrophy of the left heart.

Stenosis of the aorta. Mostly combined with insufficiency. Harsh systolic bruit. Long-drawn-out, slow, small pulse (28-32 in the horse). Hypertrophy, attacks of vertigo during exercise (work).

Valvular diseases of the pulmonary artery are very rare.

Termination of all valvular diseases. In chronic heart diseases the hypertrophy and dilatation of the ventricle is followed by a relative insufficiency of the valves. Semilunar defects lead to a relative insufficiency of bicuspids; bicuspid defects to a relative insufficiency of the tricuspids. The special diagnosis of the primary lesion is then very difficult. As sequela, finally, the following symptoms appear: small, irregular pulse, systolic and diastolic bruits, congestion of veins, venous pulse, edemas, dyspnea, albuminuria, dropsy, attacks of vertigo, emaciation and great weakness.

Pericarditis. Mostly a symptom of other diseases. Moderate fever, congestion of mucous membranes. Pulse rapid, heart's beat weak or imperceptible, zone of cardiac dullness increased, pericardial (frictional) bruits, which disappear when fluid exudate becomes prevalent. The pressure of the exudate upon the veins causes congestion in jugulars (venous pulse).

Traumatic pericarditis of the ox. Begins usually with the symptoms of an acute indigestion (traumatic inflammation of the stomach and diaphragm), which may continue for some time. If the pointed foreign body is driven forward, which is commonly caused by the expulsive efforts of the abdominal muscles during the act of parturition, it usually reaches the heart. The general condition of the patient is greatly disturbed, the expression complaining, anxious. The animals stand with back arched and held stiffly, do not like to lie down, and when recumbent rest continually on the sternum. When arising they utter complaints. Temperature variable, external (surface) temperature never quite normal. Pulse rapid, artery tense. Heart beat cannot be felt, zone of cardiac dullness increased and tympanitic when gas has accumulated in the pericardium. On auscultation in the earlier stages pericardial frictional bruits, heart sounds clear, when much exudate is present weak; systolic bruits of a metallic character in consequence of spasm-like contractions of the heart. When putrefactive gases are present the heart sounds can be so loud and metallic as to be heard at a distance. Jugulars distended, pulsating (undulating), edema of brisket, neck and throat. Course chronic notwithstanding severity of the ailment. Prognosis bad.

7. Respiratory Apparatus.

The examination of the respiratory tract is one of the most important responsibilities of the veterinarian, first because it is frequently subject to disease, and secondly from its availability to thorough inspection.

From the complex anatomy of the apparatus, and the value to diagnostics of the varied clinical phenomena it manifests in disease, a searching examination of the respiratory tract can only be made by following a definite system.

The examination would include attention to the following:

I. The respiratory movements (respirations).
II. The breath.
III. The nasal discharge.
IV. The nasal cavities and adjacent sinuses.
V. The submaxillary lymph glands.
VI. The cough.
VII. The voice.
VIII. The laryngeal region.
IX. The trachea.
X. The percussion of the thorax.
XI. The auscultation of the thorax.

1. The Respiratory Movements. [Respirations].

The respirations should be examined in regard to frequency, manner in which produced, and any special sounds originating during the act of breathing. These three factors help to determine whether dyspnea be present or not.

Frequency of respirations. To determine the number of respiratory movements per minute each rise or fall of the flanks or ribs is counted. Observing the play of the nostrils is not as certain a method, as these organs can be voluntarily moved by the animal. In winter the breath can be seen appearing as steam at each expiration. The respirations should be counted for at least thirty seconds; in restless animals the veterinarian should stand quietly near, count several times and take the average obtained as the respiratory frequency.

In birds (fowls) the respirations may be counted while the patient stands or sits quietly and unmolested, by noting the movements of the flanks and abdomen.

The smaller the animal the greater the number of respirations. In one and the same animal the number of respirations per minute will vary within physiological limits.

Just after partaking of food, or when the abdomen is very full, and especially after exercise, an acceleration of respirations is a normal consequence. High atmospheric temperatures, restlessness and anxiety, also make the breathing more hurried. In adult animals standing at perfect rest the following number of respiratory movements per minute may be taken as the average normal:

Horse	8-16
Ox	10-30
Sheep and goat	12-20
Swine	10-20
Dogs	10-30
Cats	20-30
Goose	20-25
Chicken	40-50
Pigeon	60-70

Fig. 28a.

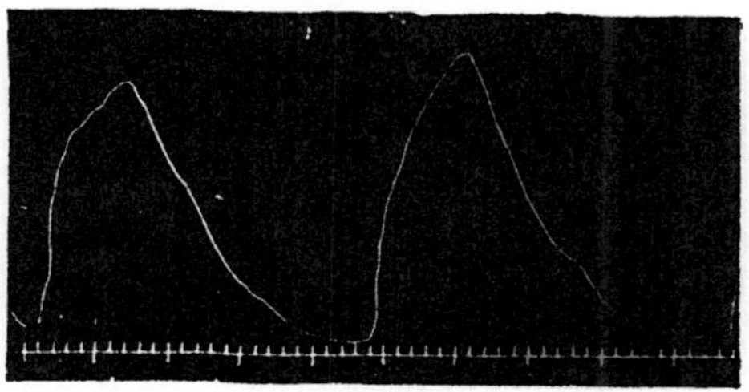

Normal Respiration Curve.

Fig. 28b.

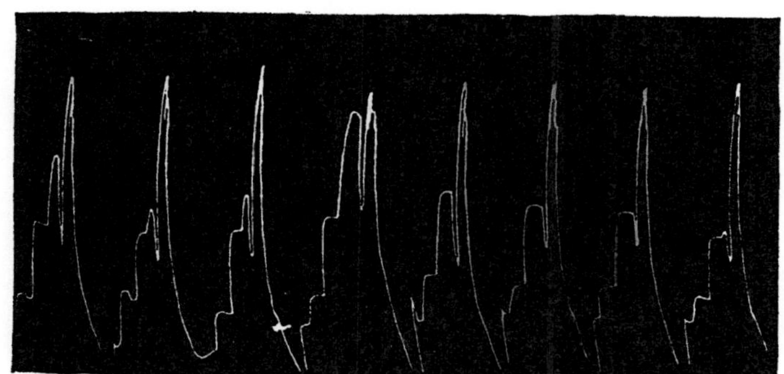

Pure Inspiratory Dyspnea in Case of Bilateral Paralysis of Larynx. The Breath Is Slowly Drawn In, Accompanied by a Strong Shaking of the Thorax.

Fig. 28c.

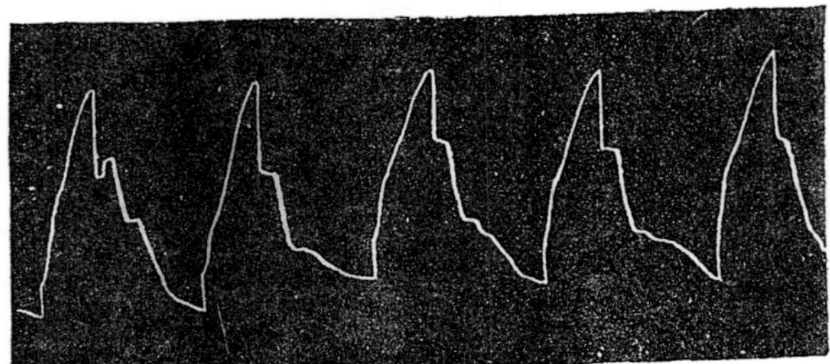

Expiratory Dyspnea in Case of Emphysema Pulmonum.

Fig. 28d.

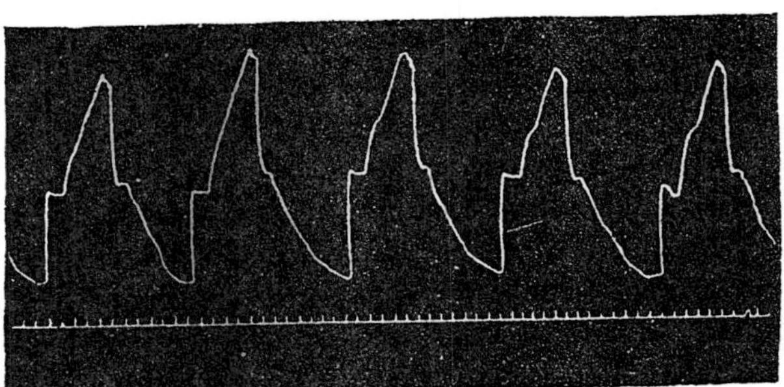

Inspiratory and Expiratory Dyspnea in Case of Inflammation of the Lungs or Thoracic Wall.

A pathological increase in the number of respiratory movements (polypnea) is spoken of as *dyspnea* (see this).

A decrease in the number of respiratory movements (oligopnea) is rarely observed. It is seen in severe brain affections (hemorrhage, hydrocephalus, tumors, poisonings, action of septic substances as in pulmonary gangrene), also where the anterior air passages are occluded (stenosis), which is combined with a pronounced inspiratory tone. Oligopnea associated with respiratory noise is always a sign of severe illness.

b. Physiology of respiration. When an animal is at perfect rest, the respirations are produced by the action of the diaphragm. The contraction of the diaphragm produces a dilation of the thorax. When the muscle contracts it flattens and is drawn backwardly, the false ribs becoming elevated. Notwithstanding that the diaphragm is stretched transversely between the thoracic and abdominal cavities, its contraction does not cause its points of insertion to approach each other, for the reason that the intestines keep it continually forward, which produces a **drawing anteriorly** of the ribs rather than to cause them to approach the median line. On account of the double articulation of the ribs with the dorsal vertebrae the forward movement of them is accompanied by a rotation. The diaphragm dilates the thorax in that it draws the ribs forward and rotates them outward at the same time.

The expiration follows the relaxation of the diaphragm, which takes place immediately after the inspiration. The duration of expiration is longer than that of inspiration; between them in quietly breathing animals there is a short pause.

1. The normal *rhythm* of the respirations can be pathologically altered in that:

The *inspiratory* movement lasts too long, the free entrance of air, being prevented by stenosis of the respiratory passages (inspiratory dyspnea).

2. The *expiratory* act lasts too long, the relaxation of the diaphragm not sufficing to a complete expiratory movement (expiratory dyspnea).

As the respirations are in a measure controllable by the will, which depends upon the cerebrum, excitement or inflammatory conditions occasioning either irritation or depression of this organ can bring about marked change in the rhythm of respiration. The value of these changes to diagnostics is limited.

A peculiar change in the rhythm and intensity of the respirations, occurring in cycles, is noted in severe intoxications and infections. It is known as *Cheyne-Stokes respirations.* Following a pause in the respirations the breathing progressively increases in frequency and intensity to dyspnea. It then slowly subsides until another pause when the cycle is repeated.

2. The *intensity* (depth) of the respirations is not marked in healthy animals standing at rest. The alae of the nostrils are hardly moved, and the ribs but slightly raised. The intensity is increased by exercise; if it is augmented and the animal at rest, it denotes disease. The horses dilate the nostrils trumpet-like, dogs open the mouth (pant) and protrude the tongue. The movements of the ribs and flanks are pronounced. The development of the intensity agrees with the degree of dyspnea.

The intensity is diminished when the pleura, chest wall or diaphragm is diseased and painful.

The intensity can become asymmetrical in that one side of the thorax undergoes a deeper or more rapid movement than the other side. This is seen in painful unilateral pneumonias or pleurites.

3. When the rhythm and intensity of breathing is normal and the ribs and abdomen are moved with even regularity, the type of the respirations is spoken of as *costo-abdominal.* if the respiratory movements are produced principally by the auxiliary muscles of breathing, which dilate the thorax, the type becomes *costal.* The costal type is seen to occur where air can not pass freely into the thorax or where the diaphragm or adjacent organs are diseased. (Abdominal tumors, ascites, tympanitis.)

When of the costal type the respirations are slow.

When the abdominal muscles are more active in producing the respiratory movement than the thoracic muscles the type of breathing becomes *abdominal.* The abdominal type prevails when painful conditions of the chest wall are present and where expiration is difficult, as in pulmonary emphysema (heaves).

4. There is sometimes observed in animals a condition corresponding to hiccoughs (*singultus*) in man. It is characterized by a rhythmic, spasmodic contraction of the diaphragm. (abdominal pulsation) with which a jerky movement of the thorax in the hypochondriac region occurs. Occasionally it is accompanied by a dull sound. Its rhythm is synchronous with neither the heart's beat nor the respirations. The latter, however, are temporarily arrested by the spasms. Singultus is usually temporary and probably due to a diaphragmatic neurosis.

C. Respiratory Sounds.

The respirations of healthy animals are performed noiselessly. Only occasionally do they voluntarily emit audible sounds during the act of breathing.

Physiological Sounds. When excited suddenly by perceiving peculiar looking objects, strange persons, unaccustomed odors, etc., horses and cattle *snort* by violently and noisily forcing air through the dilated nostrils. Horses of lively temperament usually snort when led at the end of the halter. Horses blow their noses by causing a forced expiration which is accompanied by a vacillating noise. As in man, dust or mucus is thus removed from the nasal organs. Fat, rough coated dogs *pant* when the weather is warm even when they are at rest. While performing hard work or during forced exercise the breathing is rapid and deep; the air passing in and out of the dilated nostrils at each in- and expiration produces a perceptible *puffing* sound. Spirited horses while being ridden at a gallop, emit a blowing expiratory sound every time the forefeet come in contact with the ground.

A *yawn* is a long-drawn-out, deep inspiration taken with the mouth *held wide* open. The inspiratory muscles assist in producing it.

Pathological Sounds (*stridores*). When the respiratory apparatus is diseased the following pathological sounds may occur:

1. The *wheezing* or *blowing* sound which is stenotic in its character, emanates from the nasal cavities. It is more pronounced at inspiration, and results from a narrowing of the nasal chambers due to the presence of tumors, swelling of the alae of the nostrils, septum or chonchae, enlargements of the turbinated bones or fractures of these bones, fractures of the nasal bones, or deposits of exudate on the mucous membrane. Depending upon the condition of the mucous membrane, the stenotic sound may be accompanied by either moist or dry rattling noises.

2. *"The Mucous Click"* (*klatschender Nasalton*) is a peculiar metallic, short expiratory sound first described by Dieckerhoff. It occurs during an inspiratory-expiratory dyspnea if the nasal mucous membrane is very moist. At a forced inspiration that part of the nasal mucous membrane which unites with the skin of the false nostril, is sucked against the opposite wall to which it adheres for a moment; when an expiration takes place this adhesion is broken, causing a metallic "slapping" tone to be emitted. This sound is of no significance.

3. *Sneezing* is an explosive expiration through the nose, which originates reflexly from irritations to the nasal mucous membrane. It is heard in rhinitis (nasal catarrh) or when foreign bodies enter the nasal cavities. Sneezing only occurs in the dog, cat, and fowl.

4. *Snoring* takes place when the act of breathing is effected through the open mouth, the soft palate undergoing a fluttering motion. In swine and dogs it occurs when the lumen or the nasal cavities is contracted by swelling or thick-

ening of the mucous membrane. Snoring is also noted in the ox when the retro-pharyngeal lymph glands are swollen or enlarged; further in the course of parturient paresis. Horses under chloroform sometimes snore.

5. *Rattling* is a stenotic laryngeal sound which occurs when the vocal cords are relaxed. It is heard in severe inflammations of the larynx or of the neighboring pharyngeal mucous membrane; phlegmon of the pharynx and edema of the glottis.

6. The most important pathological respiratory tone is the *stenotic laryngeal tone.* Normally the sound emitted by the larynx is a soft stenotic sound audible when the ear is placed over the organ. [It can be imitated by pronouncing the German "ch"]. If the lumen of the larynx is narrowed, the noise becomes loud. It is most frequently heard in the horse, and is one of the characteristic symptoms of roaring.

Ordinarily the tone is emitted when the respirations are increased during exercise, but in cases where the lumen of the larynx is much diminished, it may appear when the patient is at rest.

The character of the tone will vary from *whistling* to a pronounced hoarse or *roaring* sound.

Besides it may be due to a firm swelling of the laryngeal mucous membrane (phlegmonous laryngitis, strangles), tumors in the larynx or its neighborhood which prevent the free entrance of air.

7. *Loud rattling noises* [garglings] are heard when the larynx or the trachea contains loose masses of mucus.

8. *Groaning* (*moaning, grunting*) is heard when a long inspiration is followed by a prolonged, audible expiration through a partially closed glottis. The sound is emitted only at expiration. Groaning is not necessarily a sign of disease, for it often occurs in healthy animals, especially cattle after a full feed or when pregnant. Groaning is produced by the

pressure of the distended abdominal organs upon the diaphragm, shortening the expiratory moment, which the animals seek to retard by partially closing the glottis.

d. Labored Breathing, Dyspnea.

The collective term dyspnea is applied to essential deviations from the normal in the frequency and kind of respiratory movements, and the occurrence of accompanying pathological sounds.

Physiologically a dyspnea occurs whenever the blood flowing through the respiratory center contains an abnormal amount of CO_2. Accordingly, anything which increases the quantity of CO_2 in the tissues, or interferes with the exchange of gases in the lungs, can cause a dyspnea.

Clinically the presence of dyspnea is recognized:

I. If the respirations are *accelerated* (altered in number), and the increased frequency is not attended with change in the manner of breathing the *dyspnea* is *simple*.

In the horse, for instance, the number of respirations can exceed 80-100 per minute and be superficial, only the nostrils becoming dilated.

If the dyspnea is severe, however, the intensity of the respirations is increased.

Simple dyspnea appears:

1. In fever; the degree of respiratory frequency depends upon the severity and nature of the disease.

2. In all conditions which make the respiratory act painful: diseases of the pleura, diaphragm, thoracic wall, peritoneum.

3. Where the breathing surface of the lung is decreased or where the organ is prevented from properly expanding: pneumonia, pulmonary tuberculosis, abdominal tympanitis, ascites.

4. In diseases of the heart which have a congestion of the blood in the lungs as a consequence.

II. If the respirations are labored (altered in quality), though the frequency may be normal, *aggravated dyspnea.* The occurrence of respiratory noises always indicates a difficulty in breathing. Depending upon whether the expiration or inspiration is difficult, an *expiratory* or *inspiratory* dyspnea is distinguished.

The inspiratory dyspnea. If the entrance of air into the respiratory organs is made difficult, the animal seeks to overcome the condition by taking forced inspirations. Not only is the diaphragm actively employed, but other muscles which are normally not used during inspiration are called into play. These muscles are: the serratus magnus, serratus anticus, external intercostals, levatores, costarum, scalenus. The following clinical symptoms characterize dyspnea:

The nostrils are widely distended; dogs fowls, cattle and swine breathe with their *mouths open.* Dogs sometimes close the jaws and breathe through the lateral commissures of the mouth, sucking in the cheek at each inspiration. The head and neck are extended horizontally, the larynx is retracted, the ribs greatly elevated and rolled forward. The forelimbs are spread far apart and the elbows turned out so that the serrati and pectoral muscles can better come into play.

If, in aggravated inspiratory dyspnea, the air enters the lung very slowly, notwithstanding that the ribs are greatly elevated, and the thorax is distended to a degree which does not correspond to the quantity of air passing in, a suction pressure will occur, which can be recognized by a *sinking of the lower anterior thoracic wall*—particularly of its intercostal spaces.

Inspiratory dyspnea is observed:

1. In a pure form in bilateral paralysis (paraplegia) of the larynx and in severe cases of unilateral paralysis of the organ (hemiplegia, roaring). It is characterized by the above cited inspiratory dyspnea and the occurrence of a stenotic laryngeal bruit. In less severe cases of roaring this symptom can only be brought out by exercising the patient. The act of expiration is performed without difficulty.

2. In less pure form where a stenosis of the nasal passages, pharynx, larynx or trachea exists due to inflammatory swellings, tumors, etc. In such cases a stenotic sound is emitted at each inspiration and the expiration is more or less difficult.

3. In diseases of the bronchi and lungs preventing the free entrance of air: bronchitis, pulmonary edema, pneumonia.

4. Where the principal respiratory muscle, the diaphragm, is inactive: rupture or inflammation, tympanitis.

Expiratory dyspnea appears when the exit of the air from the lung is made difficult. In this case the expiration ensues not alone passively, but the accessory expiratory muscles actively assist. The muscles aiding expiration are: the abdominal muscles (external and internal oblique, straight abdominal muscle), the internal intercostals and triangularis. An expiratory dyspnea is recognized by the following symptoms: The expiration is prolonged and is attended with pronounced movement of the abdominal wall (*pumping of the flanks*). At first, a limited sinking of the thoracic walls ensues from a relaxation of the diaphragm, then the abdominal muscles become active (contract) and a furrow is formed along the course of their insertion to the costal cartilages—the so-called *"heave line."* The passive and active moments of expiration can be plainly distinguished from each other, so that the movement of the flank appears to be a *double pump-*

ing. The back is elevated at expiration and sinks during inspiration. At the moment of expiration the *anus* is greatly *protruded.* When the abdomen is well filled, these symptoms appear more prominently.

Expiratory dyspnea occurs:

1. In vesicular and interstitial emphysema.
2. In chronic bronchitis and peri-bronchitis.
3. Where the lung has adhered to the costal wall.

A mixed dyspnea is present when accelerated respiratory frequency is combined with difficult inspiration and expiration (*inspiratory and expiratory dyspnea*). It is the most common form of dyspnea and attends all severe diseases of the respiratory tract (pneumothorax, hydrothorax) and also those diseases which haye no primary seat but whose course is accompanied by a severe intoxication of the blood with CO_2—as in many of the infectious diseases.

In pronounced mixed dyspnea there is a marked flapping of the nostrils. At the beginning of inspiration both wings (medial and lateral) are greatly distended. At the end of the inspiratory movement they again collapse. However, the forced out-flow of air at expiration, which immediately follows, forces the medial wing, which is in its path, outward and upward causing a second movement of this wing to occur.

According to the seat of the respiratory obstruction one speaks of a *nasal, laryngeal, tracheal* and *pulmonary* dyspnea.

II. The Breath.

An examination of the exhaled air is of diagnostic importance in many morbid conditions. Normally the air is emitted from the nostrils in two odorless currents of equal size. The two deviations from the normal are: e:

1. *The air currents from both nostrils are not of equal size.* Where one of the currents is smaller (of less volume) than the other, it points to a narrowing of the nasal

passage of that side. Not infrequently a *blowing* sound accompanies the inspiration. The passages may be constricted by thickenings or swellings of the mucous membrane or by tumors.

2. *The breath has a bad odor.* A bad odor from the nostrils is always a sign that putrid decomposition is taking place in the air passages. It may emanate from various parts of the respiratory tract. The odor is either *putrid* (*fetid*) or *carious.* It is observed:

1. Where stagnant masses of putrefying exudate are in the turbinated bones, sinuses, gutteral pouches, or even on the mucous membrane of the upper air passages and bronchi.

2. In putrid decomposition of tumors in the air passages.

3. In suppuration or necrosis of the bones of the head bordering on the air passages: Suppuration in the tooth alveōli, dental caries, necrosis of the turbinated bones.

4. In gangrene of the lungs.

It is always important to determine where the odor originates. At first we should be clear as to whether it really comes from the nose or from the mouth. When the mouth is closed, this is usually not difficult; in doubtful cases the odor of the saliva can be tested. The safest way is to make an examination of the buccal cavity, especially of the teeth. When the alveoli of the upper molars are diseased, a carious smell is emitted from both the mouth and nose. (See Examination of the Mouth).

If the offensive odor has been found to come from the expired air, it is then necessary to locate the part of the respiratory apparatus at which the decomposition is taking place. For this purpose we should first determine whether or not the odor is equally offensive from both nostrils. When the odor from one nostril is more prevalent than from the other, the process of decomposition has its seat in the nasal cavity of that side, and usually it is accompanied by a unilateral nasal discharge, bulging of the facial bones and swelling of the submaxillary lymph glands.

The examination of the upper molar teeth of that side should never be neglected.

When the odor is equally offensive from either nostril, the putrid focus is as a rule contained in the lung, more rarely in the pharynx, larynx or trachea.

Putrid decomposition in the lung is not always to be ascribed to pulmonary gangrene, for not infrequently a decomposition of exudate in the bronchi, (*fetid bronchitis*) is present.

The presence of elastic fibres in the nasal discharge speaks for pulmonary gangrene.

III. Nasal Discharge.

Only in the ox a slight nasal discharge is seen to occur in health, which the animal usually removes from the nostrils with its tongue. In the other animals the appearance of a nasal discharge is always a sign of disease, and one of considerable diagnostic importance. It can accompany all diseases of the respiratory tract which are exudative in character, such as catarrhs of the nasal cavities, sinuses of the head, throat, larynx, trachea, bronchi and lungs. In these cases the discharge is the product of the disease. Sometimes the discharge comes from the digestive tract, from the mouth or pharynx, more rarely from the gullet or stomach, when it contains substances such as food particles, water or saliva.

The character of the nasal discharge depends upon the organ from which it comes and the nature of the disease producing it. We should bear in mind that the ox, sheep, goat and dog usually lick off the discharge, hence it is not so noticeable in these animals as in the horse.

To correctly judge nasal discharge the following should be considered:

a. The quantity, which will vary greatly. The discharge is *slight* in catarrhs that are neither very diffuse nor severe. In tuberculosis, notwithstanding the severity of the case, there is little discharge because what little exudate appears upon the surface of the mucous membranes is removed by coughing and eventually swallowed.

The discharge is *copious* in strangles and in diffuse catarrhs of the upper air passages and bronchi.

Unilateral nasal discharge is characteristic of disease of one side of the anterior air passages as far back as the fauces. A catarrh involving but one side of the soft palate or pharynx may also show a discharge from only one nostril.

Of especial importance is the *variation in quantity* of the discharge. In some cases a copious amount of discharge is ejected when the head is suddenly lowered [unreining after a drive], while for a day or more there is present either no discharge at all or only a very slight one. This symptom is characteristic of catarrhs of the frontal and superiormaxillary sinuses and of the guttural pouches.

b. The color. The color of the nasal discharge depends upon the character of the inflammation, and also the presence of foreign mixtures. It will vary from *colorless* to *grey, white, yellow, red, brown* or *green* in all their different tints. During the course of a disease the color of the nasal discharge will change with the character of the inflammation. A serous or mucous discharge is usually colorless; a purulent discharge is grey or yellow or may be of a greenish hue.

A *colorless* and *clear* discharge is noted in serous and mucous catarrhs.

A *gray* discharge is due to the admixture of epithelial cells; if leucocytes appear in it the color is *greyish-white;* if red blood corpuscles are present a *greyish-yellow* or even *yellow* color is given to the discharge.

A *green* discharge is usually due to an admixture of the

chlorophyll of the food, deglutition being difficult. Food particles are always present in such cases. In rare instances a greenish tinge is seen, due to decomposed blood coloring matter being present in the discharge.

A *yellow, rust-colored* ["prune juice"] discharge is seen in hemorrhagic hepatization of the lungs (contagious pleuropneumonia of the horse). It is due to an admixture of blood coloring matter.

In rare instances a rusty brown nasal discharge is present in severe catarrhal affections of the anterior respiratory passages (strangles, pharyngitis).

A *bloody* discharge (*epistaxis*) is observed only when blood *in toto* is present. It may be due to:

1. Finger-nail injuries to the mucous membrane of the nose or fractures of nasal bones. In the dog the presence of *pentastomum tenioides* may lead to bloody nasal discharge, and in sheep the larvæ of œstrus ovis.

2. Ulcers; glanders; bleeding tumors in the nasal cavities.

3. Nasal hemorrhages may attend anthrax in the ox, purpura hemorrhagica, or very severe cases of contagious pleuropneumonia of the horse.

The discharge may consist entirely of blood, or simply of an admixture of blood. If the hemorrhage is from a nasal cavity, it is unilateral, the blood appears fresh and incompletely mixes with any other discharge present. If from the lungs, it is more or less foamy and in the trachea one may hear moist rales.

c. **The consistency** of the nasal discharge depends upon what it contains. It may be *serous, mucous* or *mucilaginous,* with varied intermediations. It may also be *flocculent, clumpy,* or contain great *masses of adhering exudate.* In the beginning of a catarrh the discharge is serous (clear), but by admixtures of mucus it becomes mucous and loses its transparency from the quantity of epithelial cells it contains. Its color is then grey. When an admixture of pus is present the discharge assumes more of a *cream-like* consistency and its color changes to greyish-yellow or yellow. A discharge of pure pus only occurs when an abscess ruptures into the nasal cavity.

A clumpy, buttermilk-like discharge is observed in chronic catarrh of the sinuses of the head because the exudate has been retained for a time.

Adhering masses of exudate are seen in diphtheritic, croupous, or fibrinous inflammations.

d. The odor. The odor of the nasal discharge becomes *foul, putrid* or *carious* from decomposing processes. In such cases the breath is also tainted. For the determination of the seat of the disorder, what has been said concerning the odor of the expired air applies.

e. Foreign admixtures. Most commonly we observe *air bubbles* of large or small size which cause the discharge to appear as foam.

Fine foam. When the discharge comes from the smaller bronchi in pulmonary edema and bronchitis, the foam is composed of small air bubbles of equal size. When there is much foam the discharge is white in color. Horses suffering from chronic bronchial catarrh after exercise show a white nasal discharge partially made up of fine foam.

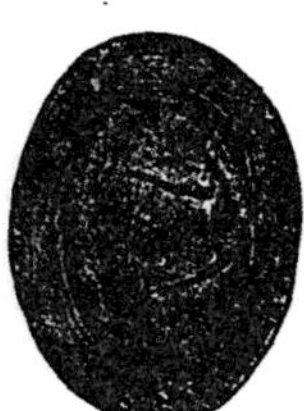

Fig. 28. Egg of Pentastomum Tenioides.

Coarse foam. This is not infrequently unilateral and contains an admixture of *food particles.* It comes from the mouth and consists in part of saliva. The air bubbles are of unequal size. Coarse foam is symptomatic of paralysis of the pharynx, pharyngitis (fungus poisoning).

When food particles alone make up the nasal discharge, it is a sign that vomiting has taken place. The discharge is then not foamy, is of acid reaction and contains no admixtures of exudate.

A microscopical examination of the nasal discharge is rarely of practical value. It may sometimes be of use to determine the presence of the embryo or egg of Strongylus filaria in the lungs of sheep or of Pentastomum taenioides in the nasal passages of the dog, or in fetid nasal discharge, the elastic fibres.

The examination for pathogenic microorganisms yields positive results only in exceptional cases. The tubercle bacilli are one of these exceptions as their characteristic way of accepting stains serves to identify them microscopically.

Microscopical determination of tubercle bacilli. A cover-glass preparation is covered with Ziehl's carbolized-fuchsin solution (fuchsin 1, absolute alcohol 10, carbolic acid 5, aq. dist. 95), and heated repeatedly for about two minutes over a flame. Wash and drain. Gabbet's solution (methylen blue 2, in 100 grammes of a 25% sulphuric acid) is then applied and allowed to remain ½ minute. Wash and examine.

Fig. 29.

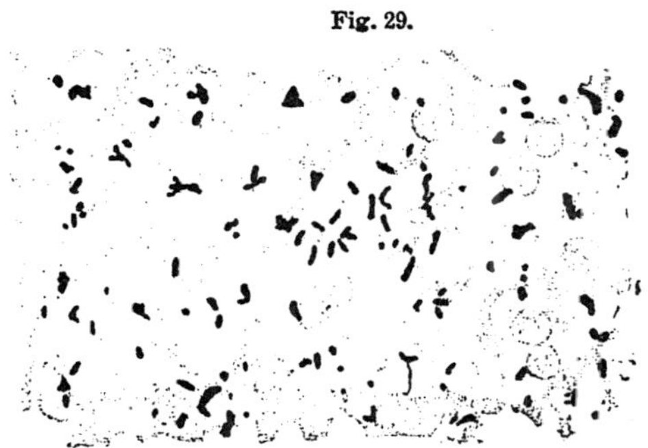

Tubercle bacilli.

Besides the tubercle bacillus, other bacilli (*acid-fast*), which stain by this method, are found in the feces of cattle and in butter.

IV. The Nasal Cavities and Adjacent Sinuses.

1. The external appearance of the facial bones will readily betray any deformity. *Circumscribed enlargements* are due to tumors and a bulging of the sinuses in chronic catarrhs. *Diffuse enlargements* attend rachitis and osteoporosis, "big head." *Depressions* have a traumatic origin. Swellings appearing at the nasal openings and nostrils are common in pupura hemorragica. Tumors (atheromas) are frequent in the false nostrils.

The specific pathological conditions which occur about the lips and nose are the *pustules* and *ulcers* which attend contagious stomatitis, the *pox pustules* of sheep pox, and the *vesicles* on the muzzle of the ox and snout of swine suffering from foot and mouth disease.

When a nasal discharge has existed for a long time, the integument of the nose and lips over which it flows loses its pigment. The white streaks thus formed speak for the chronicity of the discharge.

2. The examination of the nasal mucous membrane. The nasal mucous membrane is available to inspection only in the horse. Local lesions occurring on it are often of great diagnostic importance.

Method of examination. The head of the animal should be elevated and the inner cartilaginous wing of the nostril grasped between the thumb and middle finger which draws it upward and outward; the extended index finger is then inserted under the outer wing, which it distends. The patient should face the light, except when the rhinoscope (an enlarged ophthalmoscope) is used.

a. Discolorations. *Indistinct, punctiform,* or *ramiform redness* is not infrequently seen in acute and chronic catarrhs; they are due to the peculiar anastomosing of the capillaries and are of no diagnostic value.

Deep redness is mostly the result of hemorrhages in the mucous membrane. They appear mostly punctiform and can be as large as a ten-cent piece, they are well circumscribed and of round form (*petechiae, ecchymoses*). When they become confluent, the redness is diffuse or appears in irregular streaks. Petechiae are most commonly seen in purpura hemorrhagica, but may also occur in severe anemia (rare) and in leucemia. The spots, which are at first dark red, soon fade and assume a brownish hue. Suffusions are observed in septicemic diseases: anthrax, septicemia.

b. **Swelling** of the nasal mucous membrane is characterized by the normal surface of the mucous

Fig. 30.

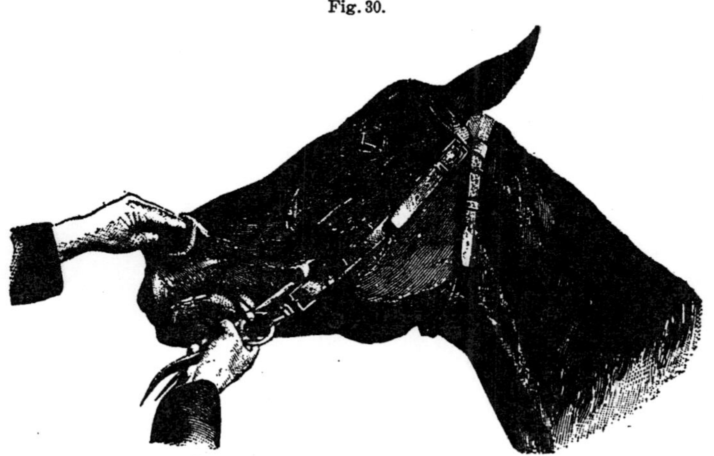

Examination of the Mucous Membrane.

membrane, which is granular from the many glands it contains, becoming firm and smooth. As the membrane is usually tense, the swelling is not marked. Its origin is inflammation, therefore the surface appears turbid.

Chronic, connective tissue thickenings are most commonly made manifest by irregular, wart-like prominences which show the characteristics of scars.

c. **Wounds in the mucous membrane** are usually at the lowest part of the septum, and are very often caused by finger-nails, sharp straws and the like.

d. **Nodules** from the size of a millet seed to that of a peppercorn almost exclusively attend glanders. Exceptionally they result from contagious stomatitis, but in such cases like nodules are to be found in the mucous membrane of the mouth. To prevent mistaking particles of mucus for true nodules, the supposed nodule should be palpated with the finger; if mucus particles, we can thus wipe them off.

e. **Ulcers.** Next to nodules, ulcers form the most important criterium in diagnosing glanders. Glanders ulcers have jagged borders circumscribed by rounded, elevated walls. The base of the ulcer is sunken, uneven, grey in color, and of lardaceous appearance. The favorite seat of the glanders ulcer is on the medial border of the inner cartilaginous wing of the nostril, hence this place should always be examined.

In rare cases ulceration of the nasal mucous membrane also attends stomatitis and purpura hemorrhagica. For differentiation the concomitant symptoms must be considered, such as ulcers on the buccal mucous membrane, petechiae, etc.

Very superficial pittings with sharp borders — not rounded nor red colored — represent the catarrhal or *erosion* ulcer.

f. **Cicatrices** at the lower end of the nasal septum are mostly the result of previous wounds. They are often curved ((as if made with a finger-nail. Glanders cicatrices are as a rule more or less star-shaped.

g. **A narrowing of the nasal passages** and the presence of tumors may be determined by the use of a hard rubber sound such as is furnished with the Polansky-Schindelka laryngoscope. [An ordinary urinary catheter serves the same purpose.] The sound should be passed beyond the posterior nares. In thorough-breds the nasal cavities are usually larger than in coarsely bred horses. Wherever there is unilateral nasal discharge and wheezing, blowing respirations present, the nose should be sounded.

3. **The examination of the sinuses of the head** is often of importance and should be made whenever a chronic nasal discharge exists, especially when attended with an unilateral bulging (enlargement) of the facial bones. Mere enlargements can be defined by palpation. The presence of exudates in the sinuses can sometimes be determined by percussion. The normal percussion sound of the sinuses is full, but when they are filled with exudate or tumor masses, it becomes flat. When the sinuses are only partially filled the percussion sound is not changed. Negative results from percussion, therefore, do not exclude the presence of exudate.

[A simple method of exploring the sinuses of the head, to determine whether exudate (pus) is present in them or not, is to bore a small hole into them with a "Yankee" drill. If the sinuses contain pus or other exudate, the bit becomes soiled by it and, if the contents are fetid, will smell.]

V. The Submaxillary Lymph Glands.

Although these glands do not properly belong to the respiratory apparatus, the examination of them is significant in the horse. In this animal especially, the glands become sympathetically diseased when pathological conditions exist within the domain of their lymph vessels.

Anatomy. The lymph vessels from the nostrils to the ethmoid bone carry their lymph to the submaxillary glands, a small glandular packet as broad as and a little longer than a finger, lying on each side of the intermaxillary space. They begin at the point where the inferior maxillary artery passes under the ramus of the lower jaw, and extend forward to the angle of the chin where each unites with its fellow of the opposite side. Each lobule is of about the size of a small bean. In horses of coarse conformation the intermaxillary space is often filled without the glands being swollen.

As soon as an absorption of irritant or infectious substances [bacteria] takes place in the region drained by the lymph vessels of the submaxillary glands, these organs become secondarily diseased. The primary disease usually has its seat in the mucous membrane of the nasal passages or sinuses. An examination of the glands, therefore, is of great significance in determining the pathological condition of these mucous membranes.

In making the examination the following points are to be considered:

a. Is **one** or **both** glands enlarged? In acute infectious catarrhs the glandular swelling is generally *bilateral;* in glanders frequently *unilateral,* and in tumors in the nasal passages, bad teeth and chronic catarrh of the sinuses, it is, as a rule, unilateral.

b. **Size** and **form** of the glandular swelling. Many or a few of the lobules may be enlarged to the size of a bean, pigeon or hen's egg, depending upon the primary disease in the mucous membranes. Acute swellings are *smooth;* chronic swellings lobulated (nodular), which is especially marked in glanders.

Well marked, clearly defined, smooth enlargements of individual lobules are observed in leucemia (a hyperplasia), and when malignant tumors are developing in the glands.

c. **Consistency** of the swollen glands. The swelling is *soft* in serous, *tense* and *firm* in cellular infiltration of the glands. Acute diffuse swellings (strangles) often lead to suppuration (abscess), which can be determined by *fluctuation.* In glanders diffuse abscess formation never occurs in the glands; only rarely does a small purulent focus (farcy bud) appear in the skin over the gland. Firm, hard enlargements are always due to some chronic irritation and consist of connective tissue proliferations. Such attend chronic glanders, catarrhs and dental fistulae.

d. **Temperature** and sensitiveness. When the glands are hot and tender (inflamed), the morbid condition is acute (strangles). If the enlargement of the gland is firm, cold and painless, it points to glanders, chronic catarrh, tumors or hyperplasias [leucemia].

e. **Movability of the glands.** If the irritation is chronic and attended with the formation of new connective tissue, the process involves the environing tissue, forming adhesions with its neighborhood. In acute purulent inflammation of the glands there develops in the vicinity, namely, directly beneath the skin, an *inflammatory edematous* and later a *phlegmonous swelling.*

The extirpation of a diseased lymph gland is recommended where glanders is suspected. Its object is the patho-anatomical or bacteriological examination of the gland. The operation can be performed on the standing animal when local anesthesia is employed, and is not dangerous.

VI. Cough.

Cough is a sudden expulsion of air from the lungs, following a deep inspiration. The glottis is forcibly opened during the act, causing a sound to be emitted. By coughing accumulations of mucus are removed from the bronchi, trachea or larynx. In animals cough is a reflex action which can to a certain extent be suppressed. Although it can be induced by irritation to many peripheral nerves, as a rule it emanates from branches of the vagus nerve in the respiratory apparatus. Most sensitive in this particular is the superior laryngeal nerve, which is the sensory nerve of the larynx, and the first three rings of the trachea. The mucous membrane of the trachea is less sensitive, except at the bifurcation of the bronchi. The bronchi are just as easily irritated as the larynx; but cough can not be excited from the parenchyma of the lungs. It can, however, arise from the pleura when this organ is in a state of irritation. Peripheral irritation is transmitted to the cough-center in the brain, which innervates the expiratory muscles and recurrent nerve, inducing the reflex spasm called cough.

In exceptional cases cough can emanate from terminals of the vagus nerve lying outside of the respiratory apparatus, as, for instance, from the external auditory meatus [ear], nose, or abdominal organs. According to Albrecht cough can occur from abscess in the liver. These are, however, exceptional cases. Cough from the stomach has never been observed in the horse. There is a possibility that cough may have its origin in the brain. These exceptions are worthy of note and should be considered in those cases of cough the cause of which cannot be found to lie in the respiratory apparatus.

Cough occurs:

1. If foreign bodies are inhaled: smoke, dust (dusty food), acrid gases (ammonia, sulphurous acid, chlorine, etc.).

2. If cold air is inhaled, especially if the respiratory tract is inflamed: catarrhs of the trachea and bronchi, pleuritis, traumatic injuries to the pleura (traumatic gastro-diaphragmitis of the ox).

3. If mucus, exudate or foreign bodies (food) and parasites are present in the air passages: Gastrus larvae in the larynx, Syngamus trachealis in the wind pipe, Strongyli in the bronchi.

In no case can cough originate when the sensory terminals of the vagus nerve are no longer susceptible to irritation. In severe phlegmonous diseases of the mucous membrane, cough is absent. The cough center in the brain must also be in normal condition. It is disturbed when great mental depression exists. Therefore, when appreciable irritations (rales) are present, unaccompanied by cough, the prognosis is an unfavorable one.

The character of the cough. The character of the cough varies with the species of animal. Healthy horses have a *strong, vigorous, loud, full-toned* cough; cattle a sharper defined, *softer, toneless, prolonged cough,* the glottis being held open. The appearance of cough in animals is always abnormal; its character depends upon the disease which causes it. Whether cough accompanies the disease or not can usually be learned from the anamnesis, although we can not depend upon this to determine its character. It is always best that we induce the patient to cough in our presence; this may be done by pinching the upper three rings of the trachea or pressing the finger ends of both hands against the arytenoid cartilages of the larynx. In sensitive healthy horses one or a few short coughs will follow the manipulation, while in indolent individuals there is no reaction.

Healthy cattle can not be made to cough by simply pinching the trachea, and even those with diseased lungs may fail to react. A better method is to close both nostrils for a minute, which usually has the desired affect.

If the ox can be made to cough by pinching the upper trachea or larynx, or if coughing takes place in the horse when only slight pressure has been used, some abnormal irritation exists. If cough can be readily induced by pressing the lower windpipe, a tracheitis is present.

The **frequency** of the cough. A cough may be *occasional* or *frequent, continual* or *transitory.* If the cough is occasional usually only one or a few impulses occur, but when frequent several in succession—a *fit of coughing.*

The **painfulness** of the cough is recognized by the general behavior of the patient, which seeks to suppress the pain by shaking the head and making masticatory and swallowing movements. The animal may also be restless, paw and groan. A *painful, painless, burdensome,* and *torturing* cough may be distinguished. The cough is painful in acute bronchitis, pleurisy, pleurodynia, and in so-called "whooping cough" of dogs; painless in chronic laryngitis.

The **force** of the cough impulse depends upon the vigor of the action of the expiratory muscles and the elasticity of the lungs. Accordingly, the cough may be *strong, vigorous,* or *weak.* It is weak if expiration is difficult or if the patient is unable to cough vigorously: reduced, debilitated animals, pulmonary emphysema, bronchitis, hydrothorax; or if the expiration is painful: pleurisy, pneumonia, pleurodynia. The cough is strong if the elasticity of the lungs is normal and no pain attends the act.

The **length** of the cough is determined by the force with which the pulmonary air is held repressed by the closed glottis. If the pressure is great, the glottis will be suddenly forced open and the cough will be short. If the glottis is not completely closed (paralysis of the arytenoid cartilage—roaring) or the repression of the air causes pain (pleurisy), the cough is *long—prolonged.*

The **depth** and **magnitude** of the cough depend partly upon the force and duration of the cough impulse. The magnitude is influenced by the quantity of expelled air. We speak of a *deep* and a *shallow* cough.

The **cough sound** is dependent upon the force of the cough impulse, the tension of the vocal cords and the special condition of the surface of the mucous membrane. The sound may be *loud, low, clear, dull, sharp, whistling, dense, hollow, loose, moist, dry.*

The cough is moist when easily movable masses of mucus are collected below the larynx; it is dry when either no exudate is present or only small, viscid accumulations are in the air passages.

The "**return sound**" of the cough (Hustenrueckstoss). Each cough is followed by a short, deep inspiration. If the glottis is not fully open at the moment this inspiration takes place, the air rushing in causes the partially stretched vocal cords to vibrate, causing a harsh, short, laryngeal stenotic sound to be emitted. It is heard in paralysis of the larynx (paraplegia, hemiplegia) and in severe inflammatory swelling.

Expectoration. The act of coughing tends to eject masses of mucus, exudate, etc., from the bronchi, trachea, and larynx. Animals do not expectorate because that which is coughed up into the throat, as soon as it reaches the pharynx, is swallowed. Sometimes, however, a part is discharged through the mouth, the lower naso-pharyngeal wall and the soft palate being forced forward by the air passing out, which leaves the opening into the buccal cavity free. The thus expectorated mass is usually mixed with mucus from the pharynx and mouth and also with food particles.

It is possible to collect "sputum" from horses and cattle for microscopic or bacteriological purposes. The method of obtaining it is to cause the animal to cough, then place a speculum in the mouth and reaching back with your hand as far as the larynx, gather the accumulated mucus in this region.

Several times in horses suffering from tuberculosis I have thus succeeded in obtaining bronchial discharge in which tubercle bacilli were found.

To obtain bronchial discharge in tubercular suspects it has been recommended to insert a tracheotomy tube and pass a swab of cotton on the end of a wire through the opening wiping the inner wall of the wind pipe down to its bifurcation. Ostertag causes the ox to cough by closing the nostrils for a minute. He then introduces a long-handled, narrow spoon between the left cheek teeth and the tongue as far back into the throat as he can reach, turns the spoon up side down, draws it back about 10 cm., then rights and withdraws it partially filled with bronchial discharge. (See also Examination for Tuberculosis.)

VII. The Voice.

Cattle suffering from nymphomania keep up an almost continuous bellowing; in advanced cases they moan loudly and constantly. At the approach of death horses sometimes utter a shrill neigh.

Change in voice is of little significance in animals. Commonly we observe a *hoarse voice* in laryngeal catarrhs.

This is most marked in dogs. In rabies the voice suffers change. In dogs affected with this disease the bark is prolonged into a long, dismal howl, the voice being at the same time hoarse. In horses a short, squealing tone is emitted.

VIII. The Larynx and Trachea.

Inspection. Enlargements in the region of the larynx are as a rule not confined to this organ, but to neighboring tissues as the pharynx, lymph glands, subcutis.

In birds the larynx may be inspected by simply opening the bill and pressing the larynx upwardly. In dogs and cats, and to a more limited extent in goats and sheep a view of the larynx may be obtained by opening the mouth and drawing the tongue forward.

Laryngoscopy.

With the aid of the laryngoscope invented by Polansky and Schindelka, the interior of the larynx may be examined directly. For the diagnosis of inflammatory conditions in the larynx this examination is of no practical value. However,

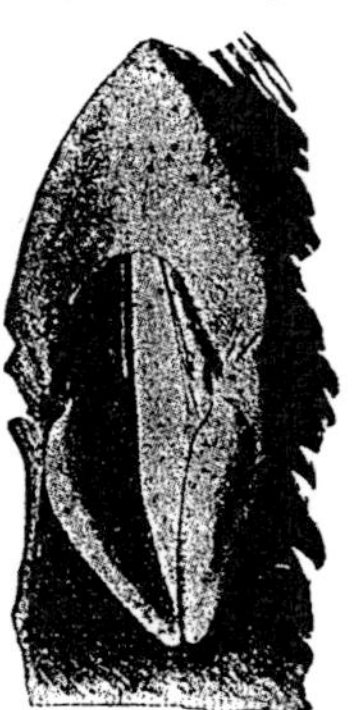

Fig. 31.
View of the larynx with paralysis of the left side, as seen through the laryngoscope.

in paralysis of the arytenoid cartilages the instrument can be used to advantage. [This instrument, which is a modified endoscope, consists of a cylinder 56cm long and 4.7cm in diameter, at one end of which is an optical illuminating apparatus. The light is furnished by an electric battery, and undue heat is prevented by a special cooling arrangement. The instrument is inserted through the nostrils and can be used in the horse without casting.] In left-sided paralysis of the larynx (roaring) the left arytenoid cartilage is seen to project farther into the lumen of the organ than the right one. This can be more distinctly seen when the larynx is moving. As the larynx of the horse is usually held in the position of "middle inspiration," it is necessary to induce forced inspiration and expiration. To do this the thorax is encircled with a girth which is slowly and gently drawn tight and relaxed, alternately, imitating forced breathing. The larynx in the meantime is watched through the instrument. At each inspiration the healthy cartilage is seen to move outwardly, while at each expiration it approaches the middle line. The diseased cartilage, on the other hand, either remains completely at rest (paralysis) or its movements are very tardily performed (paresis).

In bilateral paralysis (paraplegia) of the larynx the patient may show dyspnea when at rest—at any rate, slight excitement will induce it. In such cases one will note that both arytenoids protrude into the lumen of the larynx at inspiration; at expiration they are suddenly forced laterally and set in vibration. The paralysis can be complete or incomplete; it may not be developed to the same degree on both sides.

Palpation. When we determine the seat of the enlargements by palpation we may at the same time note their temperature, sensitiveness, and the ease with which cough can be induced by pressing upon them. Where much exudation is found in the larynx, infiltration of the vocal cords or other folds of mucous membrane, a trembling of the organ may be felt (*laryngeal fremitus*).

In examining the trachea we should look out for scars resulting from tracheotomy wounds. The form of the trachea should also be noted. In chronic tracheitis of the ox the trachea may be shaped like a saber scabbard.

Flattening of the trachea in horses is probably due to a paralysis of the transverse muscle.

On auscultation of the larynx or trachea, normally a stenotic sound is heard [like a German "ch"]. It is due to a vibration of the vocal cords and laryngeal walls which is produced by the air forced through the organ. It is heard best at expiration. When the mucous membrane of the larynx is swollen and firm, this sound becomes very pronounced and assumes a *whistling* or *hissing* character. If the swelling of the laryngeal mucous membrane is loose, or deposits of exudate cover the membrane, the sound produced is *rattling* or *purring*.

IX. Percussion of the Thorax.

To properly percuss the lungs a knowledge of their topographical position is essential.

Anatomy. The lungs and heart do not occupy the whole of the thoracic space. The abdominal viscera encroach upon a greater part of it. The partition between the chest and abdominal organs is the diaphragm. This organ is inserted, in the arc of a circle, to the inner surface of the whole thorax, reaching in an oblique direction from the sternum backwardly and upwardly to the lumbar vertebrae. In the region of the sternum its points of attachment are at the union of the ribs with their cartilages, farther posteriorly, however, the diaphragm does not extend down as far as the cartilages of the false ribs, but passes obliquely across their inner surfaces until, finally, at the last rib, it finds attachment at the superior end. The diaphragm arches forward from its points of insertion, extending into the thoracic cavity in the shape of a cone the apex of which reaches in the various animals, somewhat beyond the middle of the 7th or 8th rib. At expiration the diaphragm lies with its muscular portion directly against the lateral chest wall, the tendinous portion then forming the partition. With the beginning contraction of the diaphragm at inspiration the arch becomes flattened in that the organ is drawn away from the inner wall of the chest. The space left by the receding diaphragm is immediately occupied by the sharp borders of the lungs which then lie close to the points of insertion of the diaphragm. At the acme of inspiration the rounded, cone-like form of the diaphragm becomes more pointed and its base and apex approach each other, the ribs having been drawn forward. By this drawing forward of the ribs the transverse diameter of the thorax is increased and the base of the cone-like diaphragm broadened.

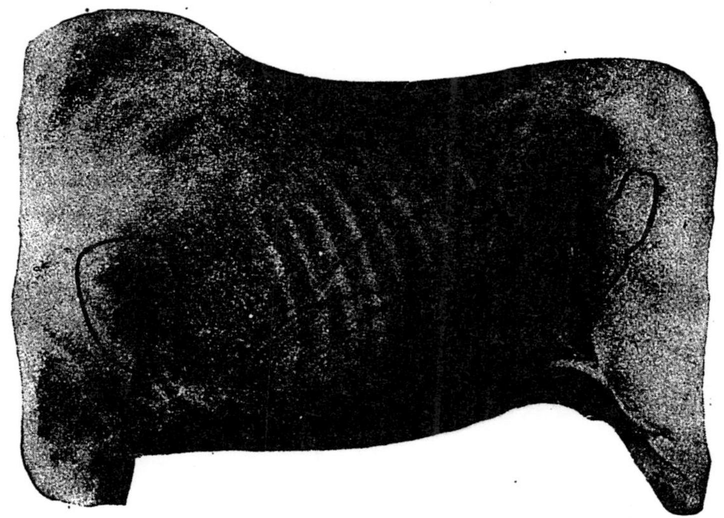

Fig. 32.

Dorsal and ventral boundaries of the field of pulmonary percussion. — - — Costal attachment of diaphram. H. heart. d. c. dorsal colon. l. v. c. left ventral colon.

Accordingly, the lateral border of the lung is continually moving backward and forward, traveling a distance in the larger animals of 1-2 hands breadth, and in the smaller ones from ½ to 1 hands breadth. On an average the posterior border of the lung may be defined by a line which in the larger animals is the width of a hand from the points of insertion of the diaphragm. In small animals the distance is one-half this.

The availableness of the lungs for clinical examination. *Dorsally* the area of percussion is defined by the thick muscles of the back. This boundary to percussion, which varies with the condition of the animal, is limited by a line drawn from the posterior angle of the scapula to the external angle of the ilium. *Anteriorly* the boundary is formed by the scapula and the massive shoulder muscles.

By drawing the leg forward the field of percussion can be somewhat enlarged. *Ventrally* the density of the sternum and muscles overlying it render in this region the lungs unavailable to percussion.

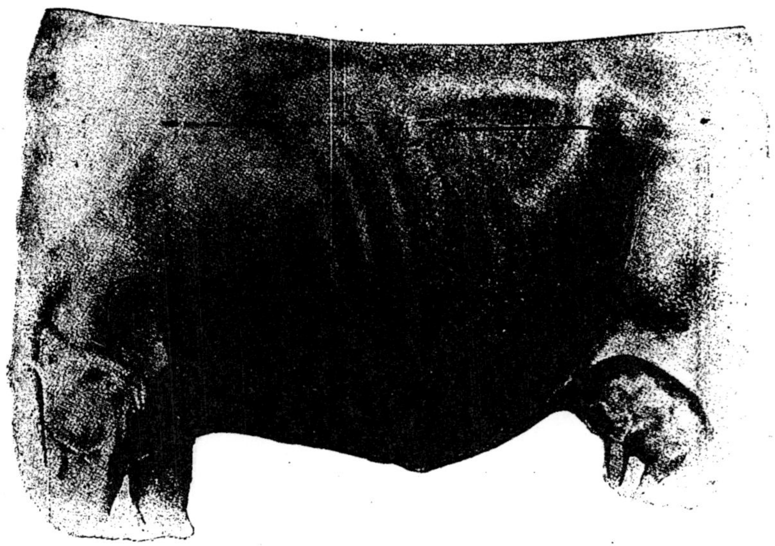

Fig. 33.

— — Dorsal and Ventral boundaries of field of pulmonary percussion. — - — Costal attachment of diaphragm. — - - — Curvature of diaphragm in median plane. - - - - Anterior boundaries of stomach divisions. H. Heart. P. Paunch.

The *field of percussion* is a right-angled triangle the right angle of which lies at the base of the scapula. In all animals the dorsal and anterior boundaries of the field of percussion are the same, the only variation being in the *abdominal boundary.*

Horse. The abdominal boundary is a line drawn from the 16th intercostal space, crossing the middle of the thorax at the 11th rib, to the olecranon.

The vortex of the diaphragm lies slightly above the of the thorax at the 8th intercostal space.

Ox. In ruminants the field of percussion is small on account of the less number of ribs (13), which causes the diaphragm to lie farther forward.

The abdominal boundary in this animal is a line drawn from the 11th intercostal space, crossing the middle of the thorax at the 9th rib, to the olecranon.

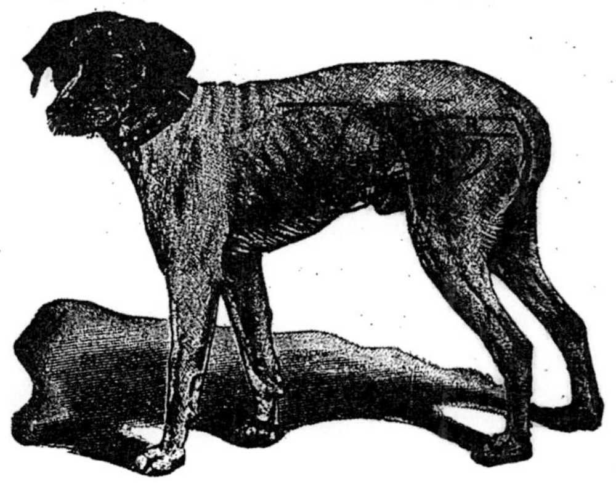

Fig. 34.
- - - - Heart, shaded portion not covered by lung. — Field of pulmonary percussion. — — — Insertion of diapragm. L. Liver. M. Spleen. N. Kidneys. R. Rectum. D. Small intestines.

Dog. In the dog the shoulder lies well forward, which gives a larger field of percussion. The abdominal boundary of the field extends at the middle of the chest wall over the 9th rib to the lower end of the 7th rib.

Swine. In swine, percussion can rarely be employed, as the thick layer of subcutaneous fat and the restlessness of the animal greatly interfere. The abdominal boundary of the field of percussion extends from the 11th rib to the olecranon.

The normal pulmonary percussion sound is due to the sound of the blow, the vibration of the thoracic wall and of the air contained in the lung. In large animals the sound is generally quite dull (subdued), but clearer in the middle and lower portions of the chest. In small animals the sound is about the same over the whole field. The thinner the chest wall, the clearer the sound. Toward the borders of the thoracic cavity the intensity of the lung sound is diminished.

The pulmonary sound is heard over an area larger than normal in vesicular emphysema, in the rarer interstitial emphysema and in pneumothorax, because in these conditions the diaphragm is forced backward. In vicarious emphysema a similar increase in area is sometimes noted.

The pulmonary percussion sound (pulmonary resonance) is abnormally loud and clear ("over-loud"), due to disease:

1. If the lung is greatly inflated (emphysema).
2. If the lung is abnormally distended with air as it occurs, for instance, at the border of pleural exudate.
3. In pneumothorax.

The **tympanitic percussion sound** is noted over the chest when the vibrating column of air, whether small or large, is surrounded by a rigid wall and there is communication with the outside world. In small animals, therefore, the pulmonary percussion sound is normally tympanitic. There is no marked boundary of distinction between the tympanitic and the full pulmonary percussion sound. A tympanitic tone is heard:

1. When a portion of the lung containing air is more or less surrounded by solidified tissue or exudate, which isolates it from its environment.

Therefore:

In the beginning and last stages of fibrinous pneumonia.

In catarrhal pneumonia.

In pulmonary edema and in pulmonary atelectasis.

In the presence of small or large tumors which surround lung containing air.

2. If caverns containing air and large bronchiectasis are present. The intensity and clearness of the sound depend upon the size of the cavern and the momentary filling of the same with air or exudate.

3. In pneumothorax.

4. In prolapse of the bowel into the thoracic cavity, through a rent in the diaphragm.

The tympanitic percussion sound has a *metallic tinkling* tone when the walls of the air-containing cavity are smooth and distended.

The cracked-pot resonance. [This resembles the sound produced by striking the hands, loosely folded across each other, against the knee, the contained air being suddenly forced out between the fingers—Loomis.] It occurs in the thorax when a large air-containing cavern is in direct communication with a bronchus. Forcible percussion causes some of the air to be suddenly driven out of the cavern into the communicating bronchus, thus inducing this peculiar resonance.

The same sound may be heard, however, when a portion of lung containing air is surrounded by a zone of hepatization. The cracked-pot resonance, therefore, does not always indicate the presence of a cavern in the lung.

If the dull or flat percussion sound is heard where the sound should be resonant, it always signifies disease. It occurs:

1. If the lung tissue becomes dense from

a. Pneumonic hepatization: in contagious pleuropneumonia of the horse, and in contagious pleuropneumonia of the ox as a rule a large portion of the lung becomes solid and liver-like, and emits, therefore, on percussion, a dull or flat sound. In catarrhal pneumonias the pulmonary sound is not so flat, because the solidification of the lung is not complete, the morbid process appearing in the form of more or less isolated centers or foci which are not entirely void of air. In hypostatic, metastatic, and ichorus pneumonias, swine plague, dog distemper, verminous pneumonia and tuberculosis the percussion sound is not diffusely dulled, but a dull sound is emitted over the dense diseased centers only.

b. Chronic interstitial pneumonia combined with atelectasis.

2. If tumors or neoformations are present in the lungs: glanders, tuberculosis, carcinoma, sarcoma, echinococci, etc.

3. If an airless, solid medium comes between the lung and the pleximeter as in;

Inflammatory swelling of the thoracic wall (after mustard applications); neoformations on the pleura; collections of considerable fluid exudate or transudate in the chest; pleuropneumonia of the horse, contagious pleuropneumonia of the ox, and in swine plague. In the horse the presence of but a few litres of fluid in the chest cannot usually be determined.

Pleuritic dullness is characterized by its *horizontal* upper boundary which shifts if the position of the body is changed, the contained fluid seeking the lowest level. This latter is most marked in small animals.

X. Auscultation of the Lungs.

During breathing, when the air enters the lung and causes it to move, sounds are produced. The occurrence and character of these sounds furnish important data in regard to the condition of the air passages and of the surface of the lung. The intensity of the sounds varies with the depth of the respirations; when the breathing is forced they are augmented. Therefore, to make them more audible it is sometimes advisable to exercise the patient before auscultating. The sounds may also be made more distinct by holding the nostrils shut for a few moments causing the patient to become dyspneic. The partial closing of the nostrils, however, recommended by some, is not admissible, as it induces a stenotic tone which might prove misleading.

a. **The vesicular murmur.** In auscultating the thorax over healthy lung, we perceive a soft, sipping sound, the *vesicular* or *alveolar murmur.* The sound can be imitated by softly pronouncing the letter "v." It begins with the inspiration, increasing as the inspiration continues, and becomes at expiration, a fainter, shorter sound, having the character of a softly aspirated letter "f."

As a rule the murmur is softer and less distinct in the horse than in the ox.

As with the laryngeal respiratory sound, so are other sounds originating in the upper air passages transmitted to the lungs. These are rattling throat sounds, wheezing, groaning, etc. Their appearance in the chest has no diagnostic significance.

An *exaggerated vesicular murmur* occurs:

1. If the respirations are intensified, therefore in physiological and pathological dyspnea.

2. If it is compensatory; that is, if one portion of the lung is required to perform extra work for another portion which is diseased and incapable of taking part in the respiratory act. [For instance, where one lung does the duty of its fellow which is diseased.]

3. If a bronchitis is setting in, the lumen of the bronchi being contracted by swelling of, or collections of exudate on, the mucous membrane. The exaggerated vesicular murmur in such cases is a symptom of great diagnostic importance.

A *diminished or feeble vesicular murmur* occurs:

1. If the thoracic wall is thickened from fat accumulations or disease: swelling, neoformations.

2. If the air cannot enter the vesicles

in consequence of great swelling or plugging of the larger bronchi: severe bronchitis.

3. If the exchange of gases in the lungs is impaired: emphysema, beginning hepatization, and a partial compression of the lungs by pleuritic exudate.

Absence of the vesicular murmur, and no other sounds present in the lung [i. e., total absence of any pulmonary sound] occurs:

1. If pleural exudates or tumors have displaced the lung tissue:

2. Rarely in severe vesicular pulmonary emphysema, or a complete occlusion of a bronchus preventing access of air into a certain portion of the lung.

Jerking, interrupted respiratory sounds are often produced by animals voluntarily, from restlessness or fear. In such cases it is heard in both lungs. Pathologically it is confined to certain portion of a lung, and is observed when the free entrance of air into the vesicles is made difficult by a contraction or occlusion of the bronchi (bronchitis).

b. **Bronchial tones.** The bronchial respiratory sound is normal in the larynx and trachea and, if the patient is dyspneic, at the root of the lung.

The occurrence of bronchial sounds in the chest is always a sign of disease. It is audible only when the bronchi are free and the vesicles contain no air.

Bronchial sounds displace the vesicular:

1. If the vesicles are filled with exudate, therefore in all pneumonias, especially in contagious pleuropneumonia of the horse and in contagious pleuropneumonia of the ox. To be heard, however, the hepatized portion of the lung must be of the size of a clenched fist and lie next to the costal wall.

2. If the lungs are compressed by pleuritic exudate (atelectasis). The compression must be complete, for if the

vesicles contain air at all a feeble vesicular murmur can still be heard.

A special variety of bronchial respiration is the *amphoric respiration,* which is a bruit like the sound produced by gently blowing across the mouth of a narrow-necked bottle. In animals it is rare, but appears if large caverns in the lung communicate with bronchi (pulmonary gangrene). On percussion, in place of the dulled sound which is usual when the respiration is bronchial, a tympanitic tone or a cracked-pot resonance is heard.

That bronchial respiration may become audible in bronchi must not be occluded; if they are filled with masses of exudate, no respiratory sound is heard. A forcible cough, however, may dislodge and eject the exudate and the bronchi become free again.

c. The vague or indefinite respiratory sounds. Such sounds are spoken of when it can not be determined whether they belong to the vesicular or bronchial respiration. Vague respiration is heard if hepatization is setting in, the vesicular murmur becoming weak and the bronchial sound just beginning. A slight compression of the lungs or partial occlusion of the bronchi with exudate may also produce it.

d. Rales or rhonchi. Rales are heard in disease and appear if the bronchi or a cavern in the lung contain movable exudate against which air is forced.

1. Moist rales appear if the bronchi contain a quantity of light, fluid exudation (bronchitis). The larger the bronchi and the greater the quantity of exudate they contain, the larger will be the bubbles and the coarser the rales. In the large bronchi and in caverns, the rales may assume a *gurgling* or *bubbling* character. We also distinguish medium, coarse, and fine rales; the latter originating in the bronchioli.

Rales may occur irregularly and are not always of like intensity. Faint rales are heard only at inspiration, increasing in intensity as the inspiration progresses; coughing may temporarily remove them. The intensity of rales depends upon the extent of the disease and the topographical position of the diseased part.

Moist rales originate from the to-and-fro movement of mucus [pus, blood, liquid exudate], the forming and bursting of bubbles, and the vibrations produced by these acts. According to whether rales attend vesicular, bronchial or amphoric respiration their tone will vary; *metallic* rales as a rule accompany bronchial respiration.

By *crepitant rales*; we understand very fine, crackling noises, which resemble the sound heard when the ear is rested very lightly upon the haired skin of an animal. Taking their origin into consideration they can be grouped with neither the moist nor the dry rales. They originate from a separation, at inspiration, of the adhering walls of the bronchi and vesicles. They appear in bronchiolitis, pulmonary edema and in the exudative (early) stage, and last stage (resolution) of fibrinous pneumonia (contagious pleuropneumonia of the horse).

2. Dry rales appear if a small quantity of a tough bronchial secretion is present, or if the mucous membrane is greatly swollen. These conditions produce more or less roughening of the mucous membrane, the projecting irregularities of which vibrate and cause sounds during in- and expiration. Dry rales are, therefore, of a sonorous, *humming*, *hissing, squeaky, whistling* (*sibilant*) character. They most commonly attend chronic diseases: chronic bronchitis, compression of the bronchi by nodules (tuberculosis, chronic pneumonia) and tumors (echinococci). In the echinococcus disease of the ox the rale has a peculiar (quurksend) character.

On account of their origin it is better to designate dry rales as stenotic sounds.

A wheezing, crackling, whistling or piping, rale-like sound is heard in interstitial emphysema of the lungs. It is most pronounced during expiration.

e. Pleuritic friction sounds. Normally the pulmonary pleura plays noiselessly upon the costal pleura during the movements of each respiratory act. If, however, the pleurae become rough and dry from inflammatory deposits upon them, a sound is produced at respiration. This sound is best heard where the movement of the pleural laminae is greatest, therefore near the sharp borders of the lung. The intensity of pleuritic friction sounds depends upon the extent of the disease [pleuritis]. They are audible as *grazing* or *rubbing sounds* just below the ear; if there is an intimate adhesion the sound is emitted in a series of *jerking, creaking,* or *crackling noises.*

A pleuritic friction sound appears in dry or fibrinous pleuritis only. It is most frequently heard in contagious pleuropneumonia of the horse and in contagious pleuropneumonia of the ox. It rarely occurs from the presence of tumors or neoformations upon the pleura. In tuberculosis, as a rule, no friction sound is heard.

Pleuritic friction sounds are easily confused with rales. **Friction sounds are heard** regularly at inspiration and expiration, may sometimes even be felt, and occur most frequently in a series of abrupt, jerking noises upon which cough has no influence. Rales are commonly more pronounced at inspiration than at expiration, are not jerking in character, and are removed or modified by cough.

Diseases of the Respiratory Apparatus.

a. Cavities of the Head.

Nasal Hemorrhage (Epistaxis.). Bleeding from the vessels of the cavities of the head. Generally unilateral. Blood appears in drops or in a thin stream and is not foamy.

Acute nasal catarrh. Rhinitis catarrhosa. Congestion of the mucous membranes, serous or mucous, rarely mucopurulent nasal discharge. Only when disease is severe is mild fever present; transient swelling of the submaxillary lymph glands.

Chronic nasal catarrh. Mostly unilateral. Discharge often mucopurulent or light colored and "glassy" in appearance; quantity varies. Nasal mucous membrane pale, sometimes catarrhal erosions. Enlargement of the submaxillary lymph glands.

Chronic catarrh of the superior maxillary and frontal sinuses. Symptoms of unilateral chronic nasal catarrh. When head is lowered discharge suddenly increases. Bulging of the diseased sinuses; if filled with exudate flat sound on percussion.

Catarrh of the guttural pouches. Rare. Usually a secondary condition. Generally unilateral, mucopurulent nasal discharge, thickening of the posterior portion of the submaxillary lymph glands, swelling of soft consistency in parotid region, which when massaged causes nasal discharge to increase. In severe cases dyspnea and dysphagia.

Tumors in the cavities of the head. Most common are sarcomas in the sinuses and polypi in the nasal cavities. Chronic nasal discharge, enlargements, wheezing respiratory sounds, submaxillary glands also diseased.

Parasites in the cavities of the head. Larvae of Oestrus ovis in the sheep, pentastomum taenioides in the dog. Sneezing, nasal discharge, wheezing respirations, brain symptoms.

b. Larynx and Bronchi.

Acute laryngeal catarrh. Laryngitis acuta. Cough which is at first dry and painful, later more moist. When disease is severe: mild fever, accelerated pulse, dyspnea with laryngeal stenotic sound.

Croupous laryngitis. Sudden fever, sometimes chills. Persistent, hacking cough. Loud laryngeal stenotic sounds, great inspiratory dyspnea.

Edema of the glottis. Suddenly appearing severe inspiratory dyspnea, loud wheezing or shrieking respiratory noise, head held extended. Stenotic sound does not disappear by partially closing the nasal openings. Peracute course.

Chronic laryngeal. Cough, especially when the animal is first brought out into the air and at work.

Roaring. Hemiplegia laryngis sinistra. An atrophy of the muscles of the larynx due to a paralysis of the inferior laryngeal nerve (recurrent), which causes an inspiratory sound. No fever, no catarrhal symptoms. Prolonged hoarse cough with return sound. Inspiratory sound when respirations are forced. Partial closing of the nasal openings causes sound to cease.

Acute paralysis of the larynx. Suddenly appearing severe inspiratory dyspnea, which is apparent when the animal is at rest or slightly excited; loud whistling or shrieking respiratory noises, anxiety, restlessness. Partial closing of the nasal openings diminishes the sound. General condition not disturbed.

Acute bronchial catarrh. May only be diagnosed when disease is well developed. Fever, accelerated pulse, dyspnea, cough which is at first dry, later loose. Full sound on percussion. On auscultation, rales which depend as to character upon the seat and quantity of the exudate.

Chronic bronchial catarrh. No fever. As a rule short, dull, weak cough. Dyspnea not pronounced at rest; at work marked. Sometimes a fine, foamy, serous nasal discharge.

Verminous bronchitis. Lung-worm plague. Develops slowly under symptoms of bronchial catarrh with prolific exudation. In mucus: parasites, eggs, or embryos of Strongylidae. Later, anemia, cachexia and death.

Strongylus filaria in sheep and goat; strongylus micrurus in ox; strongylus paradoxus in swine, and strongylus syngamus in fowls.

c. Lungs.

Pulmonary hemorrhage. Hemoptoae. Light red, foamy blood from both nostrils, cough, rales heard over trachea and bronchi.

Pulmonary Congestion and Edema. Sudden, severe in- and expiratory dyspnea, respirations may exceed 100, foamy serous nasal discharge. Percussion normal; auscultation, exaggerated vesicular sound, rales.

Pleurodynia. This is a congestion of the lungs combined with severe pains in the thoracic walls. General apathy, excessive dilatation of the thorax, which is "held." Groaning. Respirations 80 per minute, superficial. Temperature high-normal, pulse accelerated. Super-resonant sound on percussion, feeble vesicular murmur.

Catarrhal pneumonia. Bronchopneumonia. Begins usually as catarrhal bronchitis. High, intermittent fever, painful cough. Only when disease is extended can pneumonia be appreciated; circumscribed patches of dullness on percussion; vesicular murmur feeble, rarely bronchial respirations.

Gangrene of the lungs. Fever. Breath at first of a sickening, sweetish odor, later stinking. Discolored greyish-brown, tenacious nasal discharge. Percussion: tympanitic sound, cracked-pot sound; at periphery of necrotic centers, dullness. Auscultation: large rales, bronchial respiration, amphoric sound. Not infrequently combined with pleuritis.

Alveolar emphysema. May only be diagnosed when well developed. Expiratory dyspnea with "double-pumping" of the flanks, protrusion of the anus. Cough: short, dull, weak. Super-resonant percussion-sound, field of percussion enlarged posteriorly. Auscultation shows the vesicular murmur to be diminished.

Interstitial pulmonary emphysema. Suddenly appearing mixed dyspnea. Cough very superficial or absent. Super-resonant percussion sound with tympanitic accessory sound extended posteriorly. A piping sound in auscultation. Emphysema of the skin frequent.

Echinococcus disease. Ox. Diagnosis is only possible when large numbers of the echinococcus bladders are in the lungs. No fever. Dyspnea. Cough weak and blowing. Percussion dulled in patches or tympanitic. Vesicular respirations diminished.

d. Pleura.

Pleurisy. Pleuritis. Fever depending upon the character of the inflammation. Respirations accelerated and dyspneic. Frequent, painful, weak cough. Horizontal line of dullness on percussion above which a tympanitic sound is observed. Percussion will vary with the position of the body of the patient. In early stages friction sounds are heard on auscultation, later when much effusion of exudate takes place no respiratory sounds are audible.

Pneumothorax. Attends interstitial emphysema of the lungs or penetrating wounds in the chest wall. Tympanitic percussion sound in the upper portions of the thorax. Severe dyspnea.

e. Infectious Diseases Which Involve the Respiratory Apparatus.

Contagious pleuropneumonia of the horse. (Brustseuche.) [According to Hutyra and Marek, the German "Brustseuche" and what is known in the United States sometimes as "contagious pneumonia" of the horse, is the pectoral (lung and pleural) form of influenza.] This is a contagious pneumonia affecting the parenchyma of the various organs and is usually attended with secondary pleuritis. 1. Stadium incrementi begins with high fever, yellow discoloration of the visible mucous membranes, general weakness, crackling of joints. 2. Acme. Does not appear before the second or third day. Symptoms of fibrinous pneumonia with or without pleurisy, usually unilateral. Rusty brown nasal discharge, empty percussion sound with resistance under the hammer, bronchial respirations. Pleuritis: Empty percussion sound limited by a horizontal line above which is a tympanitic zone. Friction sounds which soon pass away, later no sound or bronchial respiration. 3. Stadium decrementi. The crisis appears in 7 or 8 days, temperature within 24-36 hours down to normal, all other symptoms, also pulse frequency gradually disappearing in 3 days. Complications: pleurisy, acute myocarditis. Resulting diseases: pulmonary gangrene, abscesses in the lungs, chronic pneumonia.

Scalma (Dieckerhoff) is a diffuse, infectious bronchitis with subacute course.

Tuberculosis. Tuberculosis is a contagious disease caused by the bacillus tuberculosis and characterized by the formation of very small inflammatory centers which soon undergo degeneration. The disease develops very slowly. Only advanced cases can be diagnosed by physical examination. Symptoms will vary with organ affected. Very often general emaciation.

1. Pulmonary Tuberculosis. Respirations often unchanged. Sometimes mucopurulent nasal discharge, especially after coughing. Cough regularly present. It is at first vigorous, but later becomes weak and not infrequently in paroxysms. Coughing may be induced by trotting the patient or by temporarily closing the nostrils, if it does not occur spontaneously. Percussion rarely

reveals much. Auscultation more valuable, especially after exercise: vesicular murmur exaggerated, rough; rales and vague sounds. Great tubercular enlargement of the mediastinal lymph glands induces chronic bloating.

Strangles. Coryza contagiosa is an infectious catarrh of the mucous membranes of the upper respiratory passages with secondary, purulent inflammation of their corresponding lymph glands. Begins with fever of intermittent character. Pulse at first little increased but may reach 80. Nasal discharge serous, mucous or purulent, usually bilateral and profuse. In 3 or 4 days at latest inflammatory swelling of the submaxillary lymph glands, which in 4 to 8 days later have abscesses formed in them. Pharyngitis frequently concomitant. Dysphagia, abscess formation in the subparotid and retropharyngeal lymph glands. If larynx is involved: cough, loud inspiratory noises. In old horses disease often limited to the pharynx.

Glanders, malleus is a contagious disease of solid ungulates caused by the Bacillus mallei, characterized by the formation of nodules and abscesses in the respiratory mucous membrane and skin. On the nasal mucous membrane we find gray nodules as large as millet seeds, transparent and surrounded by a red zone. The nodules become yellow, degenerate, form ulcers with raised and jagged borders and lardaceous bottom. Nasal discharge slight, frequently unilateral, varyingly sticky, slimy, purulent, occasionally discolored and bloody. Intermaxillary lymphatic glands enlarged, knotty, firm, adhering to bone or skin. In skin and subcutis rather flat, painful, hot nodules varying in size up to that of a hen's egg, these break, discharge discolored pus and become ulcerous. Lymphatics efferent and afferent to these nodules are enlarged to thickness of a finger. See also specific examination for glanders.

Contagious pleuropneumonia of cattle is a contagious, croupous-interstitial pneumonia. An occult stage is distinguished which is marked by a slight cough, fever and mild dyspnea. In the acute stage there is distinct —41 C. and the symptoms of an acute pleuropneumonia: great dyspnea, weak, short cough, slight nasal discharge, flat sound on percussion, friction bruits, bronchial sound, rales. Appetite, rumination and secretion of milk suspended.

Malignant catarrhal fever, malignant head catarrh, is a specific disease of the ox, takes a subacute course and affects chiefly the mucous membrane of the respiratory and digestive tracts. The brain is also involved. The disease is ushered in by chill; great nervous depression, muscular trembling, stiffness, sometimes inability to stand. Conjunctivitis and keratitis. Diphtheritic inflammation of the mucous membrane of the nose, sinuses of the head, trachea and mouth; breathing wheezy and rattling. No appetite; milk secretion suspended.

Swine plague, septicemia suum, is a contagious inflammation of the chest organs of swine. The clinical phases vary with severity of outbreak. The usual or **pectoral form** shows following symptoms: Fever, languor, continued grunting, loss of appetite, swelling and reddening of the conjunctiva; dyspnea, painful cough, groaning, dullness over lungs on percussion; bronchial sounds; death usually from asphyxia. The **septicemic** form shows severe general symptoms and ends in death. The chronic form presents symptoms of chronic bronchitis or catarrhal pneumonia, emaciation, and stunted growth.

Dog distemper is a very contagious disease characterized chiefly by a catarrhal inflammation of the mucous membranes. Symptoms are quite varied. Catarrhal, nervous and exanthematous forms are distinguished. The disease develops slowly. Languor, conjunctivitis, keratitis, vomiting, anorexia, nasal discharge, cough, dyspnea, tympanitic to flat sound on percussion; rales. Spasms of the whole body or of muscle groups, general muscular weakness, paralysis. Vesicular and pustulous exanthema.

Fowl diphtheria is a contagious, croupous-diphtheritic inflammation of all of the mucous membranes of the head, which sometimes attacks the comb, wattles and around the eyes, assuming the form of an epithelioma. The patients are dyspneic, the respirations noisy and performed with open beak. The course is chronic.

8. Digestive Apparatus.

Diseases of the digestive apparatus are common in domestic animals. Their diagnosis is, in some respects, far more difficult than that of the respiratory apparatus because the organs concerned are not as accessible to examination. For this reason every possible factor must receive most careful consideration. We observe these in the following order:

I. Food and Drink.
II. The Buccal Cavity.
III. The Pharynx and Esophagus.
IV. Rumination.
V. Vomiting.
VI. The Abdomen.
VII. The Intestinal Evacuations.

I. Food and Drink.

Before examining the various organs of the digestive apparatus, we must note the animal's appetite for food and drink as well as the character of these latter, also observe the way in which the animal takes its food, masticates and swallows it.

a. Appetite for Food. The appetite that an animal manifests for certain food depends in part on its palatability and in part on the degree to which the animal has become accustomed to it. This must always be borne in mind when probing for the cause of poor appetite, and hence an inspection of the food must not be neglected. Individual appetites vary widely. One horse may be a good feeder, another a poor feeder, both may enjoy perfect health. High strung horses often refuse their food after active exercise, but their appetite returns after a short rest. A change of stable or unaccustomed loneliness has a marked effect on the appetite of some sensitive horses. Of the various grains horses prefer oats and indian corn and of the grasses sweet timothy or meadow hay. Oats is by far the most suitable grain to feed a horse.

In all serious cases of disease the appetite is more or less affected, hay or straw are usually the last part of the ration refused. Defective appetite alone is never an indication of any particular disease. As a rule, complete loss of appetite is an unfavorable symptom; on the other hand, a good appetite in the course of a severe disease may be regarded as a favorable symptom.

By the term *perverted* or *depraved* appetite we mean the craving of unnatural food by otherwise healthy [?] animals. As a rule this is a very important symptom. Of course this condition must not be confounded with playfulness of young animals which gnaw at, bite and even swallow almost anything of convenient consistency and size. Thus cattle will lick at one's clothes, dogs eat blades of grass.

A craving for alkalies is pathological: e. g. straw soiled with urine and feces, whitewash, etc., on walls, wood; acids in dyspepsia.

Swallowing indigestible substances, like cloth, leather, wood, stones, and similar objects is observed in lick disease of cattle, and wool eating of sheep; in rabies the same is observed.

Desire for water depends in the first place on the amount of water contained in the feed; dry feed requiring more water than green feed; of course some water is required in both cases. Under normal conditions horses usually drink one or two large pailfuls of water per day. The demand is also affected by the amount of water given off through the skin, kidneys and intestines. Many horses are very sensitive in the matter of impure water, some even refuse "pure" water if of a different kind than that to which they have been accustomed [e. g. spring water and rain water].

The desire for water is diminished in colic and in all serious gastric and intestinal affections, *providing* no diarrhea exists; horses with acute cerebritis also refuse water. Continued refusal of water is on the whole considered as an unfavorable sign; when horses with colic drink water it is regarded as a favorable sign.

Thirst is increased in the course of various diseases:

Animals with fever like small sips of fresh water at frequent intervals.

When the crisis occurs in influenza or contagious pleuro-pneumonia of the horse, increased renal secretion and thirst go hand in hand.

Exudative pleuritis and peritonitis.

Diabetes insipidus of horses is attended with marked increase of thirst; several pailfuls are taken at a time.

Diabetes mellitus.

Gastric and intestinal catarrh [diarrhea] of dogs —attended with frequent vomiting.

b. **Manner of taking food.** Healthy horses grasp the food with their lips and pass it into the mouth, then with the aid of the tongue and cheeks it is forced between the molars. Sheep and goats do likewise. Healthy cattle grasp their food with the extended tongue, curved like a hook.

In horses the following changes are observed:

1. In inflammatory swelling of lips and cheeks as well as in paralysis of the cheeks (facial or 7th nerve), horses take up their food with their *teeth* and experience difficulty in getting it into the mouth.

2. In cerebral depression they show similar peculiarities; while drinking they may insert the nostrils below the level of the water and "masticate" it.

3. In tetanus feeding is very laborious; mastication and suction movements are impossible because the spasmodic contraction of the masseter muscles has closed the buccal cavity.

In cattle normal feeding is disturbed in inflammatory affections of the tongue (actinomycosis), this organ often becoming hard and rigid (woody tongue). Cattle thus affected grab their food like dogs.

The manner of drinking water must also be observed. Normally only dogs and cats lap their drink. When the facial nerve is paralyzed animals must insert the whole mouth into the water so that they can get it near enough to the pharynx to swallow it.

c. Mastication. The briskness with which this act is performed bears a direct relation to the palatability of the food and the appetite of the animals; healthy horses and cattle make 60-100 masticatory movements per minute.

Masticatory movements are conspicuously retarded in cerebral depression, in the course of severe fevers, and in acute and chronic hydrocephalus. The animals cease masticating for some time, seem "absent minded," and forget to eat. This often happens while the mouth is full of feed, and pieces of hay and straw sticking out of it.

Mastication is made difficult in paralysis of the facial nerve; here the food collects in large masses in the lower part of the mouth; it is also observed in tetanus or spasms of the masticatory muscles due to other causes.

Mastication is impaired and laborious when mechanical

defects of the teeth exist. Shear jaws, and irregular teeth projecting teeth, etc. The animals masticate one-sided, cautiously and "easy;" they don't masticate thoroughly, the food is "crushed and bruised" but not "ground."

Mastication is painful when acute inflammatory conditions exist in the cheeks, temporo-maxillary articulation and in the intermaxillary space as they occur in the course of distemper of horses. *Mastication* may be voluntarily interrupted. If sharp or pointed objects like nails, needles, splinters of wood, etc., are taken up with the food horses open their mouths wide and allow the contents to drop out, aiding with the tongue. They do the same thing when injuries are produced by sharp teeth or displaced teeth (alveolar periostitis); sudden pain, produced by biting on a diseased or loose tooth, produces the same effect. Horses with diseased teeth frequently drop small masses or balls of food into the manger, "quibbing." Some horses suddenly raise their head while masticating and hold it sideways, open the mouth and continue masticating in a cautious manner, at the same time making slow lateral movements with the lower jaw. Varied as the symptoms that occur in the course of different affections of the teeth may be, they all have one thing in common, they make mastication difficult and painful.

In dangerous diseases we often observe *gnashing of the teeth,* at the same time this is not a "prognostically unfavorable" sign.

d. Deglutition. Deglutition is the closing act of *feeding.* It is described as occurring as follows: The lips are closed and the jaws are set together, then the tip, the back and the base of the tongue are successively pressed against the palate and thus the contents of the buccal cavity are forced into the pharynx. By contraction of the muscles of the pharynx in front of the food mass the peristaltic motion thus inaugurated carries the bolus into the esophagus.

At the same time the pharynx is slightly raised and the pressure exerted on the epiglottis by the base of the tongue, which projects backward, closes the larynx and allows the food to glide over it. The nasal openings leading into the pharynx are closed during this act by a raising of the soft palate and a coming together of the borders of the posterior pillars of the fauces brought about by contraction of the muscles of the pharynx.

A disturbance of normal deglutition is most frequently caused by inflammatory processes in the pharynx that cause infiltration and disturb the function of the local muscles. The result is not only a *painful* condition during swallowing but the closure of the larynx or nasal cavities may be incomplete. Accordingly we may observe manifestations of pain, extended head and neck, the animals often shaking their heads. Incomplete closure of the pharyngeal openings results in food particles entering the larynx or nasal cavities and giving rise to cough, or ejections of water, saliva or food through the nostrils (regurgitation), as the case may be. The degree to which the closure of the pharyngeal openings is imperfect, bears a direct relation to the severity of the affection. In mild cases, fluid only is regurgitated, noticeable while drinking water. Later on as the case becomes aggravated, solids also pass out. When the affection is mild and restricted to one side the regurgitation may also be unilateral. Soft feed is more apt to cause regurgitation than are solid substances. An inflammatory affection of the pharynx that causes difficulties in deglutition may be primary (pharyngitis), or secondary to other diseases: distemper, morbus maculosus, anthrax.

In addition, difficult deglutition is observed in:

Paralysis of the pharynx in mycoses, parturient paresis and rabies.

Spasm of the pharyngeal muscles in tetanus.

Tumors of the pharynx; actinomycoma, lymphoma, tubercular lymph glands.

Besides the symptoms of difficult deglutition we observe in addition: salivation, foaming at mouth, ejecting food from mouth while coughing, retention and fermentation of food in mouth cavity.

Fig. 35.

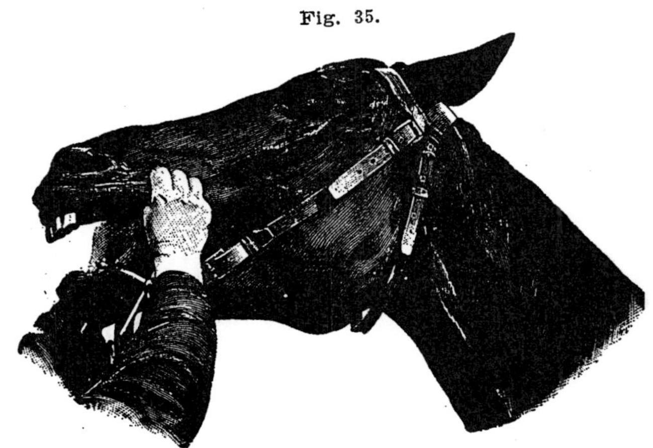

Inspection of the Mouth Cavity.

II. The Buccal Cavity.

We usually examine the buccal cavity by daylight and without the aid of instruments; artificial illumination with reflectors, lamps, or electric lights is sometimes useful but not necessary.

Method of Examination. In the horse and ox the hand is passed into the mouth at the bars, the tongue firmly grasped, and the thumb pressed against the palate. This procedure will, as a rule, cause the animal to open its mouth wide. Another practical method consists in grasping with the hands, on both sides, the upper lips at the commissures and resting the thumbs against the palate. In dogs and cats we grasp, with our hands, the upper and lower jaws, at the same time pressing the lips between the teeth; hereupon the animal opens its mouth wide enough to permit inspection.

Restless animals must first be secured and then towels or cords are passed between the dental arches, and by means of these the jaws are forced apart.

In examining the mouth the following should be observed:

The temperature is elevated in fever and in local inflammations of the mucous membrane, stomatitis and in pharyngitis.

Secretion of Saliva. Secretion is diminished in all acute febrile diseases, severe intestinal affections, and, as a rule, in colic.

An abnormal quantity of saliva in the mouth results either from the fact that the animal does not swallow the normal secretion (dysphagia) or that an abnormal secretion has occurred, as in simple catarrhal or traumatic stomatitis, diseased teeth, foot and mouth disease, stomatitis pustulosa contagiosa, malignant catarrh, mycoses, etc. The saliva passes off in the form of *clear strands* or in the form of *foam* produced by masticatory movements. In epilepsy this foam is observed at the commissures of the mouth.

Odor from the mouth. An *"insipid sweetish" odor is* observed when decomposing food-particles, epithelial cells or saliva in the course of stomatitis catarrhalis, are present. A *putrid* odor is produced by decomposition of nitrogenous substances. Exudates are present in malignant catarrh and stomacace in dogs. A *carious* odor is produced by suppurative processes in bones, especially in alveolar periostitis.

Specific morbid conditions. *Clamminess* of the buccal mucous membrane occurs in digestive disorders (loss of appetite); *reddening and swelling* of the mucous membrane with loss of substance is observed after the action of irritants and caustics [chloral hydrate pills]. Simple catarrh is attended with similar but milder symptoms.

Punctiform hemorrhages occur in morbus maculosus and leucemia. *Nodules, pustules* and *ulcers* in stomatitis pustulosa contagiosa. *Ulcers* on the gums in stomatitis ulcerosa, calf diphtheria, swine plague, mercury and lead poisoning. *Blisters* in foot and mouth disease, small isolated yellowish *vesicles* in stomatitis vesicularis. *Wounds* at the tongue tip and frenulum are produced by rough handling of the bridle bit; sharp teeth produce wounds on the inside of the cheeks, and sides of the tongue.

Foreign bodies are of frequent occurrence in horses [corn cobs], dogs, and cats, rare in other animals; they consist of pieces of bone, needles, etc., occasionally ring-like objects slip over the tongue accidentally: e. g. cross sections of the aorta, intestines, trachea, iron rings, etc., [rubber bands slipped on intentionally by children during play]. The symptoms are: open mouth and salivation, attempts at removal on part of the animal, eating and drinking interfered with, the tongue swollen.

Careful manual as well as ocular examination is often necessary to recognize these conditions.

Condition of the teeth. Examination of the teeth of horses is of particular importance on account of the frequent occurrence of diseases and malformations of these organs. In dogs diseased teeth are also common.

Abnormal position of the incisors (parrot mouth and pike mouth) point to the existence of a similar defect in the molars. Parrot mouth is not an uncommon occurrence in high bred colts. In ruminants the incisors are normally *loose*. Carious incisors and molars occur in dogs in the course of rachitis, distemper, anæmia and stomacace.

Careful examination of the molars with the aid of a speculum* is indicated when horses reject food after partial mastication, when they show any abnormal masticatory movements, and when large quantities of coarse food particles occur in the droppings. The

*[For horses a speculum is not in all cases necessary for the detection of defects or other abnormal conditions of the teeth. By passing the hand into the mouth at the bars, at the same time pushing the tongue to the opposite side that organ is forced between the molar teeth on that side and the animal will voluntarily keep its jaws sufficiently separated to permit examination of the condition of the teeth without endangering the safety of the operator. The right molars are examined with the right, the left with the left hand, the operator facing the animal.]

friction surface and the lateral faces of the teeth can be examined simultaneously by letting the index and middle fingers glide over the former, the thumb and the remaining fingers over the latter. Abnormal conditions of the teeth can usually be *felt* far better than they can be seen. We should observe the presence or absence of sharp points, slanting friction surfaces, shear jaws, *interrupted jaws*, projecting teeth, short teeth, carious and broken teeth, cavities, etc.

III. Throat and Esophagus.

Examination of the throat and esophagus is restricted to external inspection and palpation.

Inspection. Diffuse swellings in the region of the pharynx occur in phlegmonous conditions of the mucous membrane (pharyngitis). Circumscribed swellings indicate the presence of abscesses and tumors.

Palpation. Increased temperature and sensitiveness indicate acute inflammation which may be either *diffuse* (pharyngitis) or *circumscribed* (development of abscesses). The consistency is firm, yet yielding; even in abscess formation distinct fluctuation is rarely present here. Circumscribed painless swellings of firm consistency indicate the presence of tumors, usually melanosarcoma in old gray horses and actinomycoma in cattle. Palpation of the esophagus serves to detect the presence of foreign bodies, mostly observed in cattle in the form of pieces of potatoes, apples, corn cobs, etc. Esophageal diverticula and stenoses cause periodically recurring occlusions of the esophagus. Ingestion of food causes the esophagus to distend—sausage like. Such animals cease eating, or, when they attempt to eat or drink, regurgitation of the ingested mass through the nostrils takes place.

Examination with a probe or probang has no special value; the dilated esophagus, regurgitation, vomiting of food and symptoms of choking are sufficient to base upon them the diagnosis *diverticulum and stenosis,* two conditions usually coexisting. On the other hand, the fact that a probang can be passed freely through the esophagus does not exclude the presence of these conditions.

IV. Rumination.

Rumination is a specific physiological act of the digestive apparatus of ruminants. These animals feed by taking up food hurriedly and swallowing it after little or no mastication. After ingesting a sufficient amount of food in this manner, the latter, which by this time has become partly macerated by the saliva which accumulated with it in the rumen, is carefully *remasticated.* During this act the animals prefer a recumbent position. The food is forced into the mouth by a contraction of the second stomach or reticulum into which it previously passes from the rumen. Every *cud* is subjected to about 60 masticatory movements and is then *re-swallowed,* this time passing directly into the omasum and abomasum or true stomach through the esophageal groove. The whole act of rumination requires from one to two hours. When cattle are driven or oxen put to work before they had time to finish ruminating, this act is temporarily suspended to be resumed at the next period of rest.

Slight disturbances of the act of rumination can as a rule not be recognized as such.

C o n s i d e r a b l e d e v i a t i o n s f r o m t h e n o r m a l or complete suppression of rumination alone are definite signs of disease.

In the beginning disturbances in rumination due to disease manifest themselves by a reduction in the number of *cuds* chewed in a certain time, by the number of masticatory movements applied to each cud before being swallowed and by the rapidity with which the animal masticates.

The severity of the disease corresponds to the degree to which rumination is interrupted. In severe diseases rumination ceases entirely.

Rumination is disturbed in:

[All severe febrile and painful affections, surgical diseases.]

Gastric and intestinal disturbances, especially overloading and paralysis of the paunch.

Traumatic inflammation of the stomach and diaphragm.

[All cachectic diseases.]

[Many cerebral diseases.]

Eructation or belching occurs normally in ruminants only. This consists in audible expulsion of paunch gases through the œsophagus and mouth. [Eructations become distinctly audible and abnormally frequent during fermentation processes in the paunch, slight tympanitis, etc. Sometimes they are accompanied by disagreeable odors (fermentations) but the character of the food also plays a role here (onions).]

V. Vomiting.

Vomiting is a reflex (involuntary) spasmodic evacuation of the stomach or paunch contents through the mouth or nasal passages. This act is assisted by simultaneous contraction of the abdominal and inspiratory muscles. Immediately preceding the act of vomiting animals make a deep inspiratory movement. Vomiting is caused by indirect (rarely direct) stimulation of the vomiting center in the medulla oblongata.

The ease with which vomiting occurs in our domestic animals varies with the species according to the anatomical construction and the degree of fullness of the stomach. Carnivora, pigs, and birds vomit most readily and with greatest ease, ruminants less so. Horses rarely vomit. This is explained by the anatomical structure and position of the stomach. [The stomach of the horse is comparatively small and even when filled does not always come into contact with the floor of the abdomen, hence is not easily affected by abdominal contractions.]

Further, the spiral arrangement of the muscular coats, insertion of the esophagus at the *middle* of the stomach, its contracted and thickened wall at the point of insertion (in contrast to the funnel shaped thin walled structure of this organ in other animals) and the large fundus of the horse's stomach must be considered in this connection.

A vigorous contraction of the stomach will serve to overcome these obstacles and vomiting may occur in the horse. In such cases, however, there is always danger of rupture of the organ. This is the usual result when the stomach is well filled with food. Vomiting in the course of colic is therefore always a serious symptom. *If, however, the stomach of the horse is moderately filled with fluid contents, a rupture need not occur.* In such cases the act of vomiting is usually not caused by an overloaded stomach but by direct stimulation of the vomiting center. (Chloroform narcosis, hemorrhages and inflammations near the medulla).

Vomiting is always a symptom of disease and occurs under the following conditions:

During the presence of foreign bodies in the larynx or at the base of the tongue: pieces of bone, fish bones, needles, feathers, etc., also when tough, stringy mucus collects in this region in the course of pharyngitis and laryngitis.

Obstruction of esophagus.

Gastric affections, overloading of stomach, gastritis, and in certain poisonings.

Intestinal affections, such as prevent the normal progress of food masses through the lumen of the intestine and thus provoke antiperistaltic movements which cause the stomach to become distended with intestinal contents, irritation of its mucous membrane, and vomiting.

Chronic vomiting is observed in cattle and is always to be regarded as an unfavorable symptom. It indicates esophageal stenoses, diverticula, enlargement of the mediaestinal glands, hernia of the diaphragm and constriction of the pylorus.

The character of the vomited material may often serve to determine the cause of the act and the origin (stomach or intestine) of the ejected mass.

VI. The Abdomen.

Examination of the abdomen is conducted according to the following general rules:

a. Inspection. The volume of circumference of the abdomen in domesticated animals is subject to great variations and great care must be exercised here in diagnosis. For clinical purposes the size of the abdomen must always be considered in connection with the general condition of the animal, its general make up, feed, care, etc. Animals habitually kept on voluminous food in ample abundance develop a voluminous abdomen. A good plan is to inquire of the owner as to the former or usual condition of the animal in this respect. Circumscribed enlargements are usually of interest from a surgical point of view.

Abnormal distention of the abdomen may be due to:

1. *Pregnancy;* the form of the abdomen becomes barrel shaped—increasing bilaterally.

2. *Accumulation* of abnormal quantities of food in the digestive tract (in horses the cecum and colon, in ruminants the paunch and other stomachs, in dogs the stomach). In these cases the distention is due either to increased consumption of food (overfeeding) or to accumulation of food taken in normal quantities during inactivity of the bowels (constipation). In these cases the normal tympanitic tone is replaced by a dull one.

3. *The accumulation of gases* produced by fermenting food. In this case the distention is in an upward direction, the hollow of the flank is raised, and the abdominal walls become distended (tympanitis, bloat). The rapid production of gas may be due to the character of the food [legumes, crucifera, etc.] or to suspended activity of the bowels.

4. *Accumulation of fluid* (transudate and exudate) in the peritoneal cavity. This is occasionally seen in dogs, rarely

in horses. In this case the distention is in a downward direction, symmetrical and bilateral, fluctuation is observed and percussion reveals a dull area bounded above by a horizontal line. When a dog thus affected is raised to a vertical position the dull area is shifted (ascites).

5. *Tumors* in the abdomen; liver (ecchinococci and carcinoma), spleen (leukemia), glands, etc.

6. *Dropsy* of foetal membranes.

7. *Retention* of urine in dogs.

Abnormal reduction in size of the abdomen may be due to:

1. *Long continued starvation*, or, if in spite of good care, abundant food and sufficient rest an animal shows this symptom, we may conclude that lack of appetite is at fault (digestive disorders).

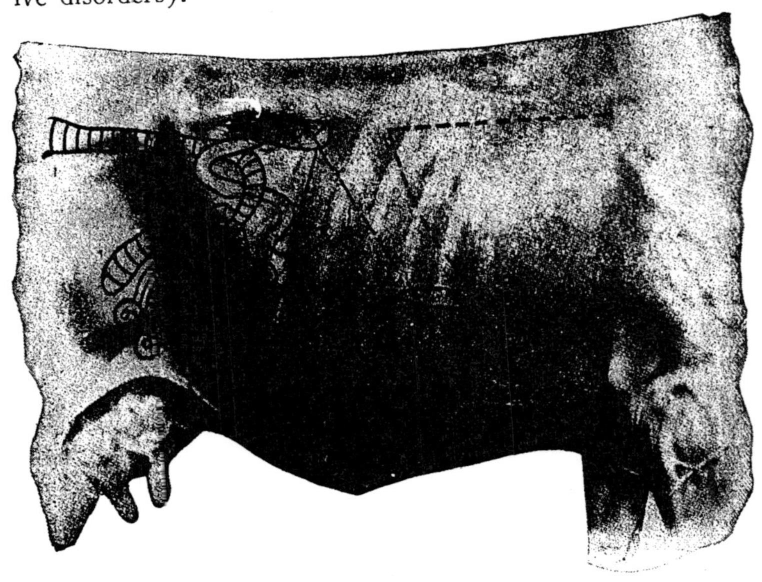

Fig. 36.

— — Dorsal and Ventral limits of area of percussion. — - — Attachment of diaphragm to ribs. N. Right kidney. L. Liver. H. Reticulum. B. Manyplies. Labm. Stomach.

2. *In serious subacute diseases;* in such cases the animal's general condition may still be good.

3. *During or following severe diarrheas,* or after colic when strong purgatives were prescribed.

4. *Violent contraction* of the abdominal muscles in painful affections of the hind legs.

b. **Palpation.** The object of palpation is to ascertain the consistency of the bowel contents and whether or not painful conditions exist. In ruminants the peristaltic motion of the bowels per rectum is of especial value in large animals.

In horses the abdominal walls are thick and tense; this and the fact that during an examination the animals frequently contract their abdominal muscles increases the difficulty of arriving at accurate results in judging of the condition of the abdominal organs, their contents, etc. In cattle the abdominal walls are thinner, hence the results of palpation are more accurate and satisfactory; in sheep this is true to a still greater degree.

Dogs habitually contract the abdominal walls when these are manipulated, but soon relax them again. In dogs both sides are palpated simultaneously, and by exerting pressure from both sides toward the median line the entire abdominal cavity may be thoroughly examined.

Palpation serves in the first place to inform us as to the degree of contraction (the tenseness of the abdominal walls and the consistency of the bowel contents; the latter should be soft and easily compressible. If impressions are made by pressure they should soon be effaced by the effects of peristalsis. Large quantities of fluid bowel contents produce fluctuation. Neoformations (tumors) are recognized by the extreme resistance they offer to pressure. In dogs accumulated fecal masses [and intussuscepted intestines] can readily be felt. Foreign bodies in the stomach and intestines can also be detected by palpation providing the normal bowel contents are previously evacuated [medicines or clysters].

Another object of palpation is to ascertain painful conditions or abnormal sensitiveness. Even healthy horses are often extremely sensitive to pressure exerted on the abdomen and become restless when subjected to such an examination. Care must therefore be observed not to mistake these symptoms for something more serious. In cattle it is different, because abnormal sensitiveness in these animals always points to the existence of important lesions.

Sensitiveness to pressure between the 6th and 8th ribs (opposite the reticulum) points to the possibility of an injury to the diaphragm from a foreign body that penetrated the reticulum. In acute affections of the true stomach cattle evince symptoms of pain on palpation of the hypochondriac region. Palpation of the right flank in cattle, when intussusception of the small intestine exists, is also attended with symptoms of pain. Foreign bodies in the intestines of dogs produce symptoms of pain when pressure is exerted.

In cattle the peristaltic movements of the paunch are an important consideration. Normally these can be felt in the hollow of the left flank at the rate of about two per minute. The food masses are moved from below upward and toward the right side. Every contraction of the paunch is attended by a slight rise in the hollow of the flank followed by a somewhat more sudden drop or depression. Imperfect or slowed movements of the paunch point to the existence of some pathological condition (overfeeding, tympanitis, paresis of the paunch, peritonitis, adhesions of the paunch with the abdominal wall).

Palpation of the bowels per rectum. This is possible only in the comparatively large rectum and roomy pelvis of the horse and ox, but on the other hand the proportions are so large here that only a part of the abdominal region can be thus explored. In the region within our reach we can determine position and contents of the abdominal organs, also the presence of foreign bodies and tumors.

Method of procedure. To make a thorough examination it is often necessary to introduce the arm full length. A shirt without a sleeve can be worn to advantage on such an occasion. [After carefully paring the finger nails] the arm should be well covered with oil, or soap (castor oil answers the purpose well) and then, with the tips of the fingers forming a cone, the hand is carefully introduced into the rectum. During the examination the animal's head (if a horse) is held up, and the forefoot on the side where the operator stands is raised, by an assistant. Nervous or excitable horses can be secured with a twitch or the operator can protect himself against kicks by having the animal standing close to a stable partition, the operator standing on the opposite side. The left half of the abdominal cavity can be examined most satisfactorily with the right hand, the right half with the left hand. Since perforations can be produced it is advisable to proceed with the utmost care in making rectal examinations.

If accumulated food masses, contraction of the rectum, or the presence of gases retard the easy introduction of the hand, simultaneous infusions of water should be given to facilitate the operation. It is always a good plan to insert the arm nearly its full length before beginning our examination. In this way a long piece of the rectum slips over the arm and there is less danger of pulling or straining the mesentery. This danger decreases as the length of the mesentery increases anteriorly.

Exploration per rectum is indicated in chronic colic and in all cases of colic in stallions and cattle. Palpation may serve to determine the following points:

I. Fullness and position of the bowels. The separate regions of the intestines can be definitely recognized only when they are filled with *food*. Mere distention with gases does not always enable us to recognize with certainty the identity of parts. When the bowels are empty or only partially filled with fluids or gases it may be impossible to distinguish between the large and the small intestine. The longitudinal muscular bands of the large intestine of the horse are the only means of differentiation, and these must be sought. Manual exploration per rectum enables us to recognize food accumulations or impactions in the following divisions of the bowels:

a. *Impaction of the floating colon.* This is of frequent occurrence in its posterior region and can then be easily recognized (rectal paralysis); constipation in the floating colon is recognized by the nodular character of the surface and the sinuous course of the bowel. Its volume is appreciably less than that of the colon or cecum.

b. *Impaction of left colon.* When well filled with impacted food masses the pelvic flexure projects into the pelvic cavity and frequently toward the right hand. This flexure is recognized by its great volume, its curvature and the short mesentery uniting the two superposed layers of the left colon.

c. *Impaction of cecum.* The base of the cecum is situated in the upper portion of the right flank and is attached to the spinal column by means of a mesenteric fold and the pancreas. When distended with food-masses its great curvature, which is smooth, projects almost to the right-hand border of the pelvis. The small curvature can also be recognized and serves to identify the organ. The longitudinal muscular bands can also be felt.

d. *Impaction of the ileum.* This usually occurs near the ileo cecal valve. The impacted intestine courses transversely from the left to the right side of the flank. It can be recognized by its sausage-like form which can be almost encircled by the hand.

The following dislocations or displacements of the intestine can be diagnosed:

a. *Incarceration in inguinal canal;* most frequently observed in stallions. The intestine can be felt about two or three inches in front of the pubic bone and four or five inches to the right or left of the median line where it seems to be firmly attached. A pull exerted at this point causes the animal to evince signs of pain. Simultaneous examination of the scrotum (external) clinches the diagnosis.

b. *Peritoneal hernia or so-called gut tie of the ox.* A loop or knuckle of intestine can be felt at the anterior margin of the ileum, retained between the latter and the vestige of the spermatic cord. The doughy, painful swelling, held in position by the tense cord which is situated anteriorly, is characteristic of this condition.

c. *Invagination of the small intestine in cattle.* This condition is recognized by the presence of a firm but elastic sausage-like mass in the lumen of the intestine, terminating abruptly posteriorly but insensibly anteriorly where food masses have accumulated. The length of this mass varies with the extent of the invagination.

d. *Torsion of the left layers of the colon* in the horse. In this condition the tense mesentery can be felt coursing downward and to the left immediately in front of the entrance to the pelvis and just below the 4th lumbar vertebra. A pull exerted on the mesentery produces symptoms of pain. A second tense strand can be felt in the umbilical region (a longitudinal band of the inferior layer of the colon which courses from left to right). The pelvic flexure has shifted from its normal position.

II. E n t e r o l i t h s (stones and concretions in the intestines) can be detected only when the intestines are comparatively empty. The presence of large masses of food interferes with their recognition. It is best, therefore, when these are suspected, to free the intestines of their contents with a purge before proceeding with the examination.

III. T u m o r s and tuberculous tumefactions of the lymphatics can be recognized only when they have a certain size, e. g., that of a hazelnut, and here too a purge must be given to remove solid fecal masses before exploration begins, otherwise mistakes are easily made.

c. Percussion of the abdomen. *Topographical anatomy.* The position of the various portions of the intestinal tract varies considerably according to their degree of fullness; we can, therefore, not define the outlines of these organs with any degree of exactness in the living animal. In a general way, however, these outlines may be defined as follows:

The right portions of the colon and the cecum occupy the right side of the abdominal cavity. We may be aided in defining the position of the various portions of the intestinal tract by drawing a line along the abdominal border of the area of percussion for the lung, and a second line along the course of the last rib and extending over the cartilages of the floating ribs; between these two draw a third (horizontal) line at the middle of the body of the animal. This outlines three areas on the right side of the abdomen. The anterior (lower) area is occupied, in the main, by the right upper portion of the colon, which occupies a position just behind the diaphragm. The ventral portion of the colon lies opposite the cartilages of the false ribs, in the region of the 8th to the 17th ribs, about half of its volume being situated above and the other half below the cartilages.

The cecum occupies the whole of the third or posterior area as well as the upper anterior area as far as the 14th rib. The small intestines and the floating colon occupy a position behind the cecum beginning at a vertical line dropped from the external angle of the ilium.

On the left side (Fig. 32, p. 125) (in the horse) the small intestine and the floating colon occupy the region of the upper two areas while the third, or lower, area is occupied by the left portion of the colon, extending up to the ilium. The lower portion of the colon occupies the greater area of the abdominal wall, the upper portion being placed more toward the median line of the abdomen, but approaching the abdominal wall as it courses forward, touching it through the medium of the diaphragm between the 7th and 11th ribs.

By careful observation of their topographical relationship, and with the aid of percussion, we can readily determine the character of the contents of the various sections of the intestinal tract.

As a rule the stomach and intestines contain a moderate quantity of gases which distend their walls *only slightly;* hence percussion produces a tympanitic sound. In the paunch of cattle and the large intestine of the horse where food masses accumulate, the sound is at times dull tympanitic or even dull. (Topography of bowels at left side in the horse; see Fig. 32.)

Abnormal accumulations of food masses in the cecum and colon give rise to a dull sound and a sensation of resistance to the finger or pleximetric hammer at points on the abdominal wall opposite them. If the accumulation of gases causes the bowel walls to distend abnormally and become *tense,* a clear sound is produced, a sound resembling that produced by the healthy lung, only clearer and louder because large air chambers are present. (In the lungs the air chambers are small).

Bilateral dullness, limited above by a horizontal line, is observed when fluids collect in the abdomen (ascites). This is most frequent in the dog; raising the animal to a vertical position shifts the dull area accordingly.

d. Auscultation of the abdomen. The observation of the various sounds produced by the moving along of the intestinal contents has for its object the determination of the character of the movements of the bowels. The sounds are produced by the onward movement of the solid, liquid and gaseous contents of the bowels. The gases particularly produce distinctly audible sounds. In the absence of intestinal contents sounds are not produced by peristaltic motion.

The character of the sounds is determined by the consistency of the intestinal contents and by the quantity of gases present. Hence: the sounds of the small intestine are those of *flowing liquid, gurgling,* and *splashing;* the sounds of the large intestine *rumbling, cooing,* and *tumbling.*

The intensity of the sounds corresponds to the intensity of the bowel movements, and we distinguish *lively, weak, hardly audible, short* and *prolonged* sounds or noise.

None of the intestinal sounds are continuous, they are always interrupted by quiet intervals, but in healthy animals

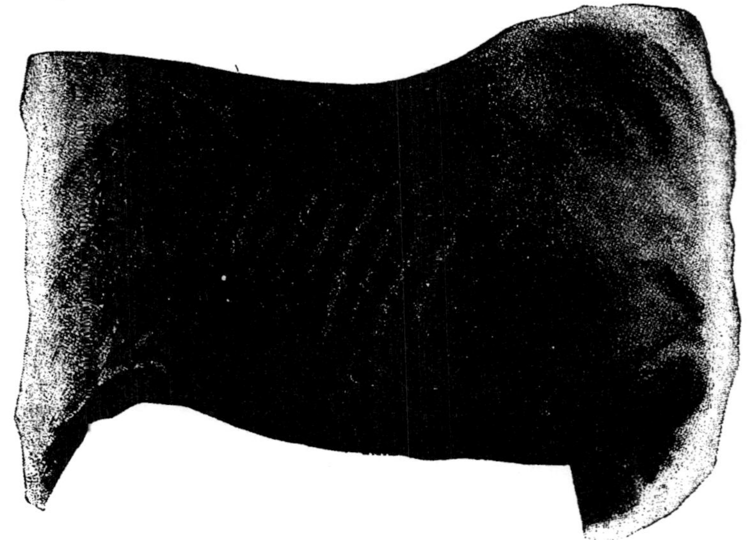

Fig. 37.

— — Dorsal and Ventral limits of area of percussion. — - — Attachment of diaphragm to ribs. Coec. Coecum. v. c. Ventral fold of the colon. d. c. Dorsal fold of the colon.

these intervals are never long. Practice in auscultation is of course necessary to enable us to judge correctly.

In disease quantitative as well as qualitative deviations from the normal occur. The sounds may be absent altogether in certain regions, e. g., the small intestine may have a lively peristaltic motion while the large intestine remains at rest.

Intestinal sounds are reduced or diminished:

In impaction, constipation and tympanitis, a paralytic condition resulting from overdistention and overloading (colic).

In spasmodic contraction of the small intestine in the course of spasmodic and rheumatic colic.

In persistent diarrhea when the intestinal contents are scanty.

In severe inflammatory conditions (because peristalsis is then more or less suspended and the intestinal contents are scanty) (enteritis, peritonitis).

Intestinal paralysis.

Very lively and loud intestinal sounds occur in all cases of slight stimulation, especially when the latter is produced by laxative food: green fodder, raw potatoes, wheat bran [clover hay, alfalfa, etc].

The sound of a drop of water falling onto a metal plate or pan is sometimes observed and belongs to a class by itself. It occurs when a loop of intestine is greatly distended and the fluid contents of the overlying intestines (small intestines) is forcibly flung against it and causes its walls to vibrate. The presence of this sound indicates that a loop of intestine is at rest and that it is distended with gas.

VII. Intestinal Discharges or Evacuations.

The quality and quantity of the discharges depend in the main on the kind and quantity of the food. The amount of water imbibed has little or no influence on the consistency of the discharges. The beginner must make an objective study of the character of the discharges of different animals on various foods, and in particular cases make comparisons with the discharges of other animals kept under the same conditions in the same stable. There are many diseases in which the character of the bowel discharges is of very great importance.

a. Defecation. The act of defecation is accompanied by an arching of the back with hind legs spread and slightly advanced; dogs assuming a crouching position. This is followed by a deep inspiration, fixing of the thoracic walls, contraction of the abdominal and intestinal muscles and relaxation of the sphinctei of the anus.

Defecation is *difficult* when the feces are dry or hard (constipation). Continued rest after and during periods of heavy feeding may lead to an accumulation of bowel contents or even to constipation. Voluntary defecation is almost impossible when paralysis of the rectum exists, in such cases the agitation of the body during locomotion causes the feces to be passively discharged through the gaping anus.

Involuntary evacuations of the bowels occur in cerebral spasms and in paralysis or relaxation of the anus. The latter is common in the course of severe diarrhœas, here the semi-liquid feces flow down on the legs.

Defecation is *painful* in the course of painful inflammatory conditions in the abdominal cavity (intestine, peritoneum), diaphragm or abdominal walls. These conditions all interfere with the normal contraction of the abdominal muscles during the act of defecation. In dogs foreign bodies (bones) in the intestines, and obstructions by agglutinated hair at the anus of long haired dogs, are particularly troublesome. The patients groan, cry or howl during attempts at defecation; they avoid the act as much as possible and thus bring on constipation.

b. Frequency of defecation. Carnivora defecate once or twice daily, herbivora much more frequently; horses 8-10 times, cattle 12-18 times. These figures are increased by bodily exercise—particularly in horses that travel much.

When the normal frequency of defecation is reduced, we say the animal is *constipated.* This is mostly the result of diminished peristaltic motion which is also attended with increased absorption of fluids. Constipation may result from impaction, occlusion, and dislocation of the intestine, first stages of intestinal catarrhs, inflammations, etc. Constipation is the principal symptom of colic, it may occur, however, without any other *colic* symptoms. In ruminants the ingesta are usually retained or retarded in the paunch and omasum, rarely in the intestines.

The term *diarrhea* is applied to frequent and usually copious evacuations of liquid or semi-liquid feces; it occurs in all irritated conditions of the intestinal mucous membrane and is caused by feed, catarrh and inflammation. Psychic disturbances may lead to diarrhea by reflex action.

c. **Volume of feces.** Here we must distinguish between the amount passed at a single defecation and the total for a day. Well fed horses (stable) pass 2 to 4 lbs. at each act, 20 to 30 lbs. per day. In acute and in chronic hydrocephalus the volume of the evacuated masses as well as the intervals between evacuations is increased. The evacuations are increased in quantity in diarrhea following constipation, they are diminished after the use of evacuants and after [prolonged diarrhea], during constipation and when animals are underfed.

d. **Consistency and form.** Under normal and usual conditions horses' dung is evacuated in balls of a regular form, which on striking the ground usually break. In cattle the dung is voided in the form of a semi-solid mass (porridge), which flattens out upon striking the ground. Sheep and goats pass small firm balls resembling the fruit of the bay-berry. Swine and dogs pass feces somewhat more solid than those of cattle and frequently quite hard. In all animals the character of the food has a great influence on the appearance of the evacuations. In describing the dung of the horse we use the terms *hard, firm, or loose balls, very moist balls, thick gruel-like mass, thin gruel-like mass, fluid, watery.*

Increased firmness or hardness of the feces is observed in all febrile diseases, in constipation, and in the first stages of intestinal catarrhs. In severe febrile diseases of cattle (malignant catarrhal fever) and in obstinate constipation the feces are dry, hard and resemble peat in appearance.

Decreased firmness or abnormal softness of the feces occurs in all forms of diarrheas, intestinal catarrh, inflammation (mycotic and septic), dysentery of calves [hog cholera], influenza of the horse, severe tubercular affections of the mesenteric lymph glands.

e. **The color of the feces** is due to admixtures of bile, coloring matter in the food (chlorophyll in herbivora, haemaglobin in carnivora) and secretions. An admixture of fragments of bone, in dogs, produces a light gray color. An exclusive milk diet produces yellow feces (bile); green fodder produces a greenish hue; oats, straw and timothy hay produce a yellowish brown color; corn, beans, rye (especially when coarsely ground) produce a gray or yellowish gray color. In cattle the diet is much more varied than in the horse, consequently it is difficult to determine a normal color. It varies from a distinct green (in pastured animals) to lighter and darker shades of endless variety. Concentrated foods (Kraftfutter) tend to produce a more grayish color.

The following morbid changes may be observed:

The longer the ingesta are retained in the intestine the darker they become. After continued constipation the feces of horses and cattle assume a blackish brown, peat-like color.

A decreased admixture of bile (icterus) produces a gray, or light gray color resembling clay. Admixtures of blood produce a red, brownish red or chocolate color, sometimes almost black. A thorough admixture of the blood with the evacuated contents points to the occurrence of a hemorrhage in the anterior portions of the intestinal tract (hemorrhagic enteritis, dysentery, etc.). If the hemorrhage occurred in the rectum the blood adheres in the form of streaks or clots.

Discolorations are produced by catarrhal and inflammatory affections. In dysentery of calves the feces are gray or grayish white. Some medicines produce *specific* colorations of the feces: iron produces a black, calomel a green color.

f. **Covering of the feces.** In herbivora the feces are covered with a thin pellicle of mucus which gives them a *shiny* appearance. This coating of mucus increases or decreases in thickness as the time during which the feces are retained in the intestine is increased or decreased. In intestinal diseases attended with extensive exudation from the mucous membrane the feces are not only coated with mucus but are mixed with it. This mucus may be glossy, colorless, yellowish (bile) or gray (epithelial cells and white blood corpuscles). Flaky or fenestrated coagulations on the surface of feces have their origin in the rectal mucous membrane (proctitis).

g. **Odor of the feces.** This varies with every species according to the food. Horse dung can hardly be said to

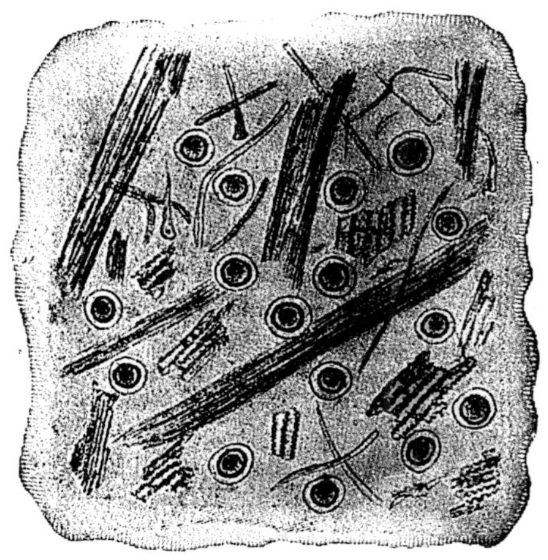

Fig. 38
Eggs of Ascaris megalocephala in dung of horse. Globular in form, diameter 0.1 mm, double contour.

have an offensive or repulsive odor, the dung of the ox has an odor peculiar to itself, and the feces of carnivora stink. Horse dung has a sour odor in digestive disorders when concentrated food was given in abundance. The feces of herbivora *stink* or have a *foul odor* when putrefactive processes go on in the diseased digestive tract. If albuminous exudates (blood) are present under these conditions the odor is carrion-like (hemorrhagic enteritis, distemper of dogs).

h. The chemical reaction of the feces has no particular diagnostic value. Horse dung, as a rule, has an acid reaction, a result of the decomposition processes going on in the large intestine. In digestive disorders and intestinal catarrhs the acidity is often increased.

i. Composition of the feces. The composition of the feces as far as food particles and foreign substances are concerned demands careful consideration. In the first place the size of the undigested food particles must be considered; this indicates the degree of mastication or rumination to which

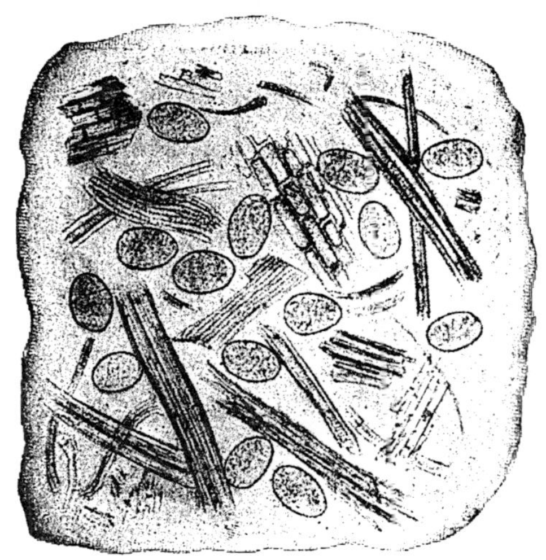

Fig. 39.
Eggs of Distomum hepaticum in dung of sheep.

they were subjected. In cattle the feces should consist of a homogeneous mass; coarse particles of food always indicate insufficient or faulty rumination: overloading of paunch, paralysis or inactivity resulting from inflammatory affections are the cause of the latter. In horses, on the other hand, coarse undigested particles of food occur normally in the dung, and faulty mastication is not indicated unless the coarse particles are very numerous and whole or nearly whole grains of corn, etc., and bits of straw or hay can be recognized. The cause of the presence of coarse particles of food consists either in greedy feeding or in defective molar teeth. The degree of the defect bears a direct relation to the degree of coarseness of the food particles.

Foreign bodies in the feces of horses usually consist of sand, and in sheep we find wool.

Inflammatory products consist of mucus, blood, pus, croupous membranes; in chronic intestinal catarrh of cattle we often find small clots of blood.

In cattle and calves suffering with catarrhs or other inflammatory conditions of the digestive tract the soft feces frequently contain numerous gas bubbles; these are due to gas-producing putrefactive organisms which are particularly active in concentrated foods that pass rapidly along the digestive tract.

Any parasites of the gastro-intestinal tract may occasionally be met with in the feces, either entire (Ascarides, Oxyuris) or in segments (proglottides of tapeworms); sometimes the eggs only are present (Distoma in sheep and cattle). When Distoma are suspected a microscopical examination of the feces should be made. The eggs of these parasites are yellowish brown oval bodies or capsules provided with a lid, (0.15mm long, 0.1mm diameter).

The most common parasites of the digestive tract are as follows:

Horse: Gastrophilus equi and hemorrhoidalis, Ascaris megalocephala, Strongylus armatus [tetracanthus], Tenia mamillana, perfoliata, and plicata.

Cattle: Amphistomum conicum, Ascaris lumbricoides, Strongylus radiatus and ventricosus, Tenia denticulata and expansa, Tricocephalus affinis, Strongylus inflatus. In the bile ducts: Distomum hepaticum and lanceolatum.

Sheep: Amphistomum conicum, Strongylus contortus,

hypostomus, filicollis and cernuus, Tenia expansa, Trichocephalus affinis, and [Tenia fimbriata]. In the bile ducts: Distomum hepaticum and lanceolatum, and [Tenia fimbriata].

Goat: Strongylus contortus, hypostomus, filicollis and venulosus, Trichocephalus affinis, Tenia expansa.

Pig: Spiroptera strongylina, Trichina spiralis, Ascaris lumbricoides, Echynorynchus gigas, Strongylus dentatus, Tricocephalus dispar. In the liver: Distomum hepaticum and lanceolatum.

Dog: Tenia echinococcus, cenurus, marginata, serrata, cucumerina, Bothriocephalus cordatus and latus, Ascaris mystax, Dochmius trigonocephalus, Trichocephalus depressiusculus.

The discharge of intestinal gases occurs only in horses and dogs; corn and green feed produce these gases in large quantities. In old cows, with chronic affections of the rectum or undue laxness of the sphincter ani, air is often sucked in during the act of expiration and expelled again at inspiration, thus producing a sound as though intestinal gases were being discharged.

Addendum. An examination of the liver and spleen of domesticated animals is usually impossible and of no practical importance because diseases of these organs are rare. As a rule, therefore, no examination is attempted.

The liver of dogs, cats and sheep will permit limited palpation only, considerable hypertrophies, tumors (carinomata) may be recognized.

In cattle the liver, if much enlarged, may be palpated per rectum and its character determined.

In tuberculosis we may recognize nodules, and in echinococcus infection recognize fluctuating vesicles.

In a horse, Marek could palpate the hyperthrophied liver at the last rib.

In cattle the liver is always accessible to percussion since it lies completely on the right side, extending from the upper end of the last rib and forming a curve ending at the lower third of the sixth intercostal space.

Since the border of the liver is thin, percussion sounds are dulled only in the field of percussion of the lining beginning at the next to the last rib and extending to the eighth intercostal space in the form of a semicircle.

Slight deviations in size cannot be determined.

The spleen is accessible to palpation in the horse only, in the upper posterior region, through the rectum.

It extends to the posterior border of the last rib.

Enlarged in leukemia, nodulated in tuberculosis.

Diseases of the Digestive Apparatus.

a. Mouth, Pharynx and Esophagus.

Stomatitis. Here the morbid changes can be directly observed; three forms: Stomatitis catarrhalis, st. vesicularis, st. ulcerosa.

Ptyalism. A continued discharge of large quantities of saliva without any assignable cause.

Actinomycosis. Multiple tumor at the lower maxilla, tongue, pharynx or adjacent regions, caused by Streptotrix actinomyces.

Pharyngitis, Angina pharyngea. More or less fever according to the character of the inflammation. Head held up, neck stiff. Appetite present but mastication and especially deglutition impaired. Food and particularly water ejected through the nose. Accumulation of saliva and food in the mouth, salivation; foreign bodies (food) in larynx, and cough. More or less symptoms of laryngitis, in serious cases dyspnea as a result of swelling of laryngeal mucous membrane.

Paralysis of esophagus and pharynx. Dysphagia paralytica, difficult deglutition and absence of inflammatory symptoms.

Foreign bodies in esophagus. Most frequent in cattle (but also observed in horses); salivation, inability to swallow, choking, flow of saliva from nose; tympanitis in cattle. Foreign body in cervical portion of esophagus can be seen or felt.

Esophageal stenoses and diverticula usually develop slowly and gradually. Symptoms: Sudden interruption in feeding, impaction of esophagus with food; regurgitation, choking. Discharged masses are foamy but not sour.

Spasm or Cramp of the Esophagus. Esophogism. Periodically spasmodic contraction of the esophagus, inability to swallow, salivation, restlessness.

Diseases of the teeth in animals produce trouble in feeding. Animals begin eating with apparent appetite, but soon stop or continue with diminished interest, masticate slowly and carefully, smack their lips, pause, salivate, reject partially masticated food, swallow their grain whole, masticate roughage poorly, don't eat a full feed, feces contain large particles of food, sometimes there is a tendency to diarrhea. The following conditons of the teeth are of clinical importance, viz., sharp teeth, very oblique grinding surfaces (shear-jaws), an undulating or irregular set of teeth, projecting or depressed teeth; caries of the teeth, tartar deposits; periostitis alveolaris, tooth fistulae, neoformations on the alveolar periosteum.

b. Gastric and Intestinal Diseases of the Horse.

Acute dyspepsia. Lack or loss of appetite, particularly for grain; animals lick cold objects. Thirst is increased, buccal mucous membrane dry, animals yawn frequently.

Acute gastro-intestinal catarrh. Usually fever, animal is downcast, conjunctiva reddened, sometimes icteric. Appetite much impaired, frequent yawning, buccal mucous membrane reddened and clammy; feces at first dry, later diarrheic; urine acid, without sediment, contains much indican.

Chronic dyspepsia. Chronically impaired appetite. Gastric disturbances.

1. Simple chronic dyspepsia. Appetite for concentrated food (grain) impaired, otherwise normal.
2. Acid dyspepsia. Impaired appetite, but a craving for alkalies; licking whitewashed walls, nibbling at soiled litter.
3. Nervous dyspepsia. This occurs in easily excitable horses and consists in temporary disturbances of appetite after excitement.

Chronic gastro-intestinal catarrh. Gastro-enteritis catarrhalis chronica. Soft consistency of feces, or hard and soft alternately, containing mucus, appetite impaired. Mucous membranes muddy red. Urine acid.

Gastro-enteritis. Inflammation of the stomach and intestine. High fever, great depression of the sensorium, mucous membranes muddy red; pulse very rapid, respiration increased. Complete loss of appetite, buccal mucous membrane hot, feces as in diarrhea, foul odor, and bloody. Rising is painful. Forms: Gastro-enteritis rheumatica, toxica, cruposa, mycotica, parasitica.

c. Gastric and Intestinal Diseases of Cattle.

Acute tympanitis. Hoven, bloat. Rapid tympanitic distention of the paunch, food and drink are refused, defecation retarded. Increased and labored breathing, animals are anxious and restless.

Acute dyspepsia. Acute derangement of activity of stomach. No fever. Feed is absolutely refused, rumination suspended, belching, abdomen full, paunch contents firm, paunch movements slight, auscultation reveals sounds of bursting bubbles, feces dry, later on containing coarse food particles.

Acute gastro-intestinal catarrh. Fever, conjunctiva reddened, pulse frequent, appetite often entirely wanting, flanks sunk in, paunch movements incomplete. Milk secretion suddenly retarded.

Chronic gastro-intestinal catarrh. Gradual development and frequent change of symptoms. Appetite reduced, bloating follows a heavy feed, rumination interrupted. Defecation usually retarded, feces mixed with mucus, now and then diarrhea. If disease is severe diarrhea is continuous. Animal weak, falls off in flesh.

Chronic tympanitis, chronic indigestion. Periodically recurring attacks of slight bloating of paunch that continue for some time. Rumination and paunch movements retarded. Coarse food particles in feces.

Dislocation of bowel. 1. Invagination (telescoping) of intestine. Occurs suddenly and without external cause. Animals are restless, lie down, get up again, kick their bellies, groan. These symptoms attended with fever. Feeding and rumination cease, obstinate constipation, discharges of mucus and blood. Pains soon grow less but fever increases. Palpation per rectum usually enables us to feel the invaginated gut.

2. Peritoneal hernia or gut tie in the ox. Symptoms same as in invagination, in addition an abducted position of hind leg which is also extended back. Sacral region depressed. Palpation per rectum reveals presence, at anterior border of ileum, of painful doughy swelling, held in place by vestige of spermatic cord.

Licking disease of cattle and **wool eating** of sheep are peculiar chronic affections; afflicted animals have a habit of licking, nibbling, or even swallowing objects of a various nature, including indigestible and often loathsome and disgusting substances. At the same time there is loss of appetite and emaciation.

d. Gastro-Intestinal Diseases of the Dog.

Acute Gastric Catarrh. Frequently febrile. Usually begins with vomiting of food masses, followed by vomiting of mucus. Loss of appetite, increased thirst, depression, evacuation of bowels retarded, symptoms of pain upon pressure over the region of the stomach.

Acute Intestinal Catarrh. Usually febrile and attended with diarrhea; feces of bad odor and frequently fermenting. Icterus and bile pigments in urine common symptoms.

Constipation. Cause, as a rule, in the rectum. Defecation retarded, animals make frequent unsuccessful attempts, tail elevated. Abdomen frequently bloated; palpation reveals impaction of rectum, painful upon pressure. Digital exploration revealing presence of hard fecal masses.

Foreign Bodies in the Intestines. Frequently situated anterior to the ileo-cecal valve. Vomiting, complete loss of appetite, absence of fever. Object can usually be located by careful palpation of pelvic region. Caution: Do not confuse with kidneys, especially in cat.

e. Diseases of the Peritoneum.

Acute Peritonitis. Usually secondary, following rupture or perforation of intestine, perforation of abscesses or extension of inflammation of adjacent organs; symptoms therefore not characteristic. Symptoms of colic, stiff gait, looking at the flank, groaning. Marked depression, staring look, moderate to high fever. Mucous membranes reddened. Pulse, rapid, small, soft. Respiration short, superficial, frequent. No appetite for food or water, abdominal muscles contracted, painful; peristalsis suspended, sometimes diarrhea as death approaches. Defecation and urination retarded, painful. Death often following after a few hours.

Chronic Peritonitis. In horses, symptoms of colic and fever, irregular appetite and emaciation. In cattle and dogs colic symptoms absent, but pain upon palpation, presence of exudates.

Traumatic Inflammation of Stomach and Diaphragm in Cattle. Indigestion of sudden appearance without apparent cause. Animals show disinclination to lie down, stand in stiff position, are very careful when rising and don't stretch. Expression of eyes indicating pain. Surface temperature irregularly distributed, bodily temperature elevated. Pulse accelerated and hard. Respiration rather retarded, groaning and manifestations of pain. No appetite for food or drink, rumination suspended. Pressure on the right side, sixth and seventh ribs, painful. Milk secretion decreased.

f. Infectious Diseases with Localization in the Digestive Tract.

Rinderpest is a readily transmissible, acute infectious disease, of cattle. It usually takes a fatal course. Period of incubation 6-7 days. High temperature is the first symptom. Eyelids swollen, conjunctiva very red, respiration difficult, dirty yellowish nasal discharge, nasal mucous membrane reddened in spots, cough, moist rales, frequently interstitial pulmonary emphysema and cutaneous emphysema; complete loss of appetite, feces fluid, discolored; secretion of milk suspended, great depression and general weakness of the body. Dark red areas on mucous membranes which (spots) become coated with grayish white layers, when the latter drop off and leave ulcerous erosions. Most animals die on the fifth or sixth day.

Calf diphtheria. Diphtheria vitulorum is an acute infectious disease characterized by compous-diptheritic accumulations on the buccal mucous membrane and caused by the Bacillus necrophorus.

Stomatitis pustolosa contagiosa is an exanthema with a typical course. It occurs in the form of pustules, principally at the mouth, and is characterized by its mild course. Period of incubation 3-5 days. At first appearance of eruption there is fever, but this soon subsides. Horses refuse feed, they salivate, mouth painful to the touch. Within 2-3 days minute nodules or blisters appear on the mucous membrane; these are at first red, then gray or yellow, break open and form ulcers. Intermaxillary glands swollen, conjunctivitis, now and then ulcers on the outer part (skin) of the lips, forearm and body; healing requires 10 days to two weeks.

Hog cholera, an infectious septicemia produced by a filterable, ultramicroscopic virus, readily transmissible. In its course multiple hemorrhages appear in the mucous membranes and skin. In the latter, superficial necrosis. At first a general febrile affection without localizations, aggravation of symptoms, conjunctivitis, red patches on the skin, often vesicular eczema and diphtherioid lesions on the buccal mucus membrane, especially that of the tongue. In the beginning constipation and bloating of the abdomen followed by excessive diarrhœa, stinking feces, drawing up and painfulness of abdomen. Septicemic, peracute cases also observed.

Swine typhus, typhus suis, a typical enteritis, not readily transmitted, caused by Bacillus suipestifer. Febrile chronic affection with progressive emaciation. Often accompanying Hog cholera and difficult to differentiate.

Dog plague (Stuttgart), typhus canum, a severe, acute, typical *contagious infectious* disease, confined almost exclusively to the digestive tract. Occurs in the form of a severe gastroenteritis and ulcerous stomatitis. Vomiting, anorexia, exhaustion, laziness, comatose condition. Never any elevation of temperature, often hypothermia.

Diarrhea of calves. Dysenteria neonatorum. A peracute infectious disease of new-born calves, resembling a septicemia. Characterized by severe diarrhea, whitish stinking feces, general weakness, and usually terminating in death within a few days.

Red Dysentery. Dysenteria coccidiosa bovum, a hemorrhage enteritis caused by coccidia.

g. Intoxications.

Lupinosis is an intoxication disease affecting the body as a whole. It is caused by a poisonous principle (lupinotoxin) which occurs in lupines. Diminished appetite, increased temperature, icteric coloration of conjunctiva, general weakness, cerebral depression. Urine yellow, contains bile pigments and albumin.

[**Loco weed poisoning.*** An intoxication disease affecting chiefly the nervous system. Effects not noticeable until a considerable quantity of the "loco weed" has been eaten. Gait slow and measured, eyes glassy and staring, vision interfered with, convulsions when animal is excited, later on, general emaciation. Occurs in western States.] *U. S. Report.

h. Diseases of the Liver.

Distomatosis, cachexia distomatosa, a disease of sheep (less frequent in cattle or goats) caused by Distomum (Fasciola) hepaticum or lanceolatum. Course chronic. The first symptoms appear six weeks, or later, after invasion of the host by the parasite. Anemia, hydraemia, cachexia. Eggs of parasite in feces.

IX. Urinary Apparatus.

In diagnosing diseases of the lungs percussion and auscultation of the chest is of fundamental importance. In diseases of the urinary apparatus we depend on the results of physical and chemical examinations of the urine. Experience has taught us that affections of the kidneys and urinary tract are not as common in animals as they are in man and consequently urinary analyses hardly merit the same importance that is attached to them by physicians. Besides this the entire field of kidney pathology in animals has received so little attention from investigators that our lack of knowledge is often evident to the diagnostician.

Results of a urine examination often enable us to diagnose affections of other organs the abnormal products of which pass over into the urine.

The collection of the urine from animals is always attended with difficulties, in practice it is often impossible. As a rule the urine is caught up in a vessel during the natural act of the animal. In horses a vessel can be secured to the sheath and the urine thus collected. In female animals the use of a disinfected catheter is permissible.

In the course of the clinical examination we consider the urine first; if the latter shows material changes we also examine the urinary organs.

Accordingly we consider the following points and in the order given:

I. Manner of Voiding the Urine.

II. Examination of the Urine.

A. Macroscopical examination.

B. Chemical examination.

C. Microscopical examination.

III. Examination of the Urinary Organs.

I. Manner of Voiding the Urine.

In our domestic animals urinating is a reflex act inaugurated by the stimulus of the urine on the mucous membrane of the distended bladder. As long as the distention of the bladder is below a certain point the reflex action of the sphincter vesicae which is also inaugurated by the pressure of the urine, supersedes that of the muscular coat, hence the one gives way to, or takes the place of, the other as occasion demands.

In adult male dogs only do we observe frequent and *voluntary* urination. For this act they prefer places used for the same purpose by other dogs. Their favorite places are trees, the corners of houses, etc.

When urine is voided the bladder contracts and this is aided by the abdominal muscles. Every species of animal manifests peculiarities of its own in this act, but it is a rule that all animals stand while urinating.

Horses (both sexes) urinate only while resting and cease feeding for the time; not infrequently they emit loud groans.

Cows urinate similarly to mares, male cattle on the other hand urinate not only while feeding but also while walking; in fact, in these animals the act *seems* almost to be a passive one.

Old dogs and pigs (male) void the urine in an interrupted jerky stream.

a. The frequency of urination depends on the amount of water imbibed, the amount of water lost by respiration, perspiration, and per intestinal tract; accordingly it varies very considerably. Healthy horses ordinarily urinate 5-6 times a day.

1. Abnormally frequent urination in usual volumes is a result of increased secretion (polyuria)

2. Diminished urination is not easily recognized in animals. In doubtful cases a clean cloth bandage may be tied over the prepuce (in the ox) to determine whether the act takes place at all. Urination is diminished or suppressed:

(a) When secretion is diminished, or when it ceases entirely (anuria) in acute nephritis. Diminished secretion is characterzed clinically by less frequent urination, continued emptyness of the bladder, concentrated and dark colored urine.

(b) When obstructions exist in the urethra (ischuria, retentio urinæ) characterized by abnormal fulness of the bladder, Concrements, swellings, strictures, tumors. Urine is passed in drops or in a thin stream often accompanied by pain.

When paralysis of the bladder exists, often accompanied by paralysis of the rectum and of the tail (myelitis spinalis). Urine is then often evacuated involuntarily during locomotion.

3. Urination is entirely suppressed in rupture of the bladder following prolonged retention of urine. Most frequent as a result of urethral calculi in wethers and steers. The urine is evacuated into the abdominal cavity. Exhalations from the body have a uriniferous odor.

b. **Abnormally frequent attempts to urinate,** only slight quantities of urine being passed at each attempt, *stranguria.* The cause of this is an abnormal irritability of the mucous membrane of the bladder and urethra. Such conditions are most frequently observed in the course of colic in horses where the distended intestines (impaction, constipation, tympanitis) exert a pressure on the bladder, or the sense of *fulness of the abdomen* causes the animals to make these attempts. Inflammatory conditions of the bladder (bladder diseases, stone and gravel, neoformations, poisoning with irritating substances) or of the urethra (applications of pepper) are much less common causes. Mares in oestrum often show these symptoms at the same time repeatedly protruding the clitoris.

c. **When urination is painful** the term *dysuria* is applied. The animals are restless, step to and fro, kick at their bellies, switch their tails, look back at the abdomen, groan, and void urine in drops or thin streams. The seat of the pain may be in the bladder or in the urethra (concrements, strictures, inflammations). Sometimes the pain is caused by abdominal pressure in *peritonitis*.

d. Retention of urine (ischury) is attended with accumulation of urine in the bladder. It is observed:

1. In obstruction of the urethra (concrements, swellings, strictures, tumors). In such cases the urine is voided in drops or thin streams, and frequently with symptoms of pain.

2. In paralysis of the bladder; frequently associated with paralysis of the rectum and of the tail.

e. Inability to retain urine, *incontinentia urinae,* occurs as a result of paralysis or weakening of the sphincter of the bladder, or as a result of diminished sensitiveness of the urethral mucous membrane, thus suspending the reflex excitability of the sphincter. Most frequently observed in dogs in the course of distemper (spinal affection) but otherwise rare in animals.

II. Examination of the Urine.

A. Macroscopical Examination.

a. The quantity of urine voided depends on the same conditions that regulate the frequency of voiding it: on the average horses secrete 4-5 liters, cattle 6-12 and dogs ¼-1 liter per day. As a rule we determine the quantity of urine voided daily by making an *estimate.* Collecting the urine for actual measurement is cumbersome and, besides, not exact.

An *increase in the quantity* of urine occurs in:

Diabetes insipidus [polyuria] (very marked) diabetes mellitus (which is rare), the daily average may be 40 liters.

Most forms of chronic nephritis.

During reabsorption of profuse exudates and in the critical stage of severe infectious diseases.

A *decrease in the quantity* of urine (Oliguria) is observed in:

Profuse sweating and diarrhea.

Severe febrile diseases.

Formation of large quantities of exudates in the pleural and peritoneal cavities.

Weak heart and resulting diminished pressure.

Acute and some forms of chronic nephritis.

b. The color. The normal pigments in urine have not yet been thoroughly studied; although a number of them are known to exist, only one has been identified, viz. *urobilin* which is a product of bilirubin and is absorbed from the intestine. The color of normal urine is more or less yellow, increasing in darkness as the amount of urine decreases, and vice versa. In disease the color may become lighter or darker. We distinguish: *yellow* (pale yellow, light yellow, yellow), *red* (reddish yellow, yellowish red; red), and *brown* (brownish red, reddish brown, and blackish brown) urine. Other shades can also be recognized now and then.

Pale, water-colored urine always occurs in polyuria (physiological or critical polyuria, diabetes).

Red urine is produced by admixture of blood, hemaglobin or methemaglobin. The particular cause in each case must be determined with the aid of the microscope.

Greenish yellow or *brownish yellow* urine or yellowish green foam is produced by bile-pigments.

Dark colored urine (dark yellow or dark brown) is observed in *all cases* where the quantity has been reduced (concentrated), but it may also be due to admixture of blood.

Color due to medicines: carbolic acid, black; aloes and rhubarb, brownish red.

c. Transparency of urine. Normal urine of the horse is always turbid; even the first few drops voided; toward the end it becomes even more so, frequently a light clay color. The turbidity is due to the presence of carbonates which precipitate in the bladder as the fluid becomes more or less condensed from reabsorption processes. When exposed to the air in a vessel the turbidity increases because the soluble acid calcium carbonate $(CO_3H)_2$ Ca after giving off CO_2 H_2O is converted into insoluble calcium carbonate CO_3 Ca. This conversion occurs most rapidly at the surface of the liquid, causing the formation of a thin fragile membrane at that place (crystals of calcium carbonate). Small granules of lime also precipitate and constitute a part of the sediment. Not infrequently these lime granules are imbedded in cylindrical masses of mucus that were molded in the uriniferous tubules. This normal *turbid* urine has an alkaline reaction.

Clear urine of the horse is always abnormal and usually has an acid reaction; upon cooling, however, it may become turbid. The turbidities consist of precipitated phosphates, oxalate of lime, and crystals of gypsum and uric acid salts; these dissolve upon heating the fluid. These salts can be recognized by means of a microscopical examination.

Abnormal turbidity may be due to the presence of organized elements (cells); recognized by means of microscopical examination.

In the ox, sheep and goat the normal urine is clear when voided but becomes turbid on standing; precipitation of monocarbonates.

The urine of the dog is clear in health, becoming slightly turbid after standing; due to precipitation of uric acid salts.

d. Consistency of urine. Normal urine of the horse is a rather thickish, slimy, viscous fluid; the viscosity being due to an admixture of mucine which occurs in the bladder. Besides this the cast off epithelial cells undergo a process of swelling and thus increase the consistency of the urine. Acid horse urine is always less viscid than such as gives an alkaline reaction because the epithelial cells swell more in the former.

All other domestic animals excrete a more watery urine.

e. **The Odor of Urine.** The freshly voided urine has an odor peculiar to each species of animal. After medical treatment with oil of turpentine the urine has an odor of violets. The odor of menthol, phenol and cresol, if given in medicinal doses, can be detected in the urine.

If freshly voided urine has a pungent ammoniacal odor, cystitis is indicated.

f. **The specific gravity of urine** is determined with an aræometer, also called *urinometer* when specially constructed for this specific purpose.

The specific gravity for the

horse	is	1020—1050,	average	1040,
ox	"	1025—1045,	"	1030,
dog	"	1020—1060,	"	1040.

The specific gravity varies inversely with the quantity. Aside from this an *abnormally low* specific gravity is observed in diabetes insipidus (1001-1010) and in contracted kidney.

An *abnormally* high specific gravity is observed in all cases where the amount of urine secreted is below the normal (fever) and in acute nephritis. *High specific gravity and increased quantity is observed only* in diabetes mellitus.

B. *Chemical Examination of the Urine.*

a. **The reaction** of the urine of healthy animals depends on the kind of food: herbivora (horse, ox, sheep, goat) secrete an alkaline urine, carnivora (dog, cat) secrete acid urine. In omnivora the reaction depends altogether on the food. Acidity increases with the nitrogen contents of the food.

In herbivora the alkaline reaction is due to the presence of acid bicarbonate of lime $CO_3H — Ca — CO_3H$.

The organic acid salts of lime which are contained in the food contain the acid radicles of malic, tartaric, succinic and lactic acids. These latter, upon being absorbed into the blood, become oxydized into acid carbonates which have an alkaline reaction.

In carnivora acid phosphates are the cause of the acid reaction; PO_4H_2Na and PO_4H_2Ca; these come from the animal diet. Starving herbivora (hence such as live on their own flesh) have an acid urine.

Except in cases like the one just mentioned an acid reaction of the urine of herbivora is always abnormal. It occurs when the contents of the small intestine have an acid reaction —intestinal catarrh. When the contents of the small intestine have a normal (alkaline) reaction the acid phosphates in the food are not absorbed, and consequently do not enter the circulation, but when the reaction is acid the opposite takes place, the acid phosphates are absorbed and excreted by the kidneys, but the *organic acid salts* are not absorbed. An acid reaction, therefore, depends on the presence of acid phosphates and, in case of herbivora with good appetite, points to the existence of intestinal catarrh.

Abnormal alkaline reaction of the urine of herbivora and carnivora occurs in the course of fermentations in the bladder (catarrh) and is produced by ammonia, which is a product of fermented urea: $CO(NH_2)_2 + 2H_2O = CO_3 (NH_4)_2 = 2NH_3 + CO_2 + H_2O$. This ammoniacal fermentation can be recognized by its odor. A glass rod dipped in hydrochloric acid and held above the surface of the urine causes fumes to appear: NH_4Cl = ammonium chloride.

b. Albumin. Serumalbumin associated with serumglobulin is the usual form in which albumen occurs in urine. Albumoses, i. e., albuminous bodies not precipitated by boiling, may be found alone or in connection with the above, but are of rarer occurrence. (Pepton, propepton, hemialbumose).

Occasionally hemoglobin and methemoglobin are found.

These three groups are alone of practical importance.

I. **Albuminuria.** Albumin never appears in normal urine in appreciable quantity; its presence must therefore always be looked upon as an indication of disease.

As a rule the albumin is secreted with the urine, in the **kidneys** (renal albuminuria), in rare cases its presence is due to admixture of blood or pathological products (accidental albuminuria).

The fact that healthy urine contains no albumin in appreciable amount is explained by the impermeability of the renal epithelium to albumin and by the limited normal blood pressure. A change from the normal, such as may be brought about by pathological conditions of the blood or increased bodily temperature, may cause the appearance of albumin in the urine.

Hence, renal albuminuria can occur:

1. As a result of *changes in the renal tissues* due to inflammatory or degeneration processes; here we find not only albumin present, but the quantity of urine may be increased by the addition of albuminous exudate.

2. *In lowering of arterial pressure*; the lower the pressure the easier can a diffusion of albuminous substances take place. Pressure is lowered in weak heart or in venous congestion (organic heart disease, emphysema). Both conditions, after existing for some time, in addition produce changes in the renal epithelium.

3. *In fever* albuminuria is always present. Several factors are active here. The lowered pressure may alone account for it; the elevated temperature facilitates the process; continued fever produces changes in the renal epithelium. In case of severe infectious fevers a direct injury to the renal parenchyma probably occurs because in such cases the urine is very rich in albumin.

4. Mere changes in the normal composition of the blood, in the absence of any change of blood pressure or change of structure of the kidneys, may bring about albuminuria (leucemia).

From what has been stated we can readily see that the mere presence of albuminuria does not necessarily indicate an affection of the kidneys.

Fig. 40.

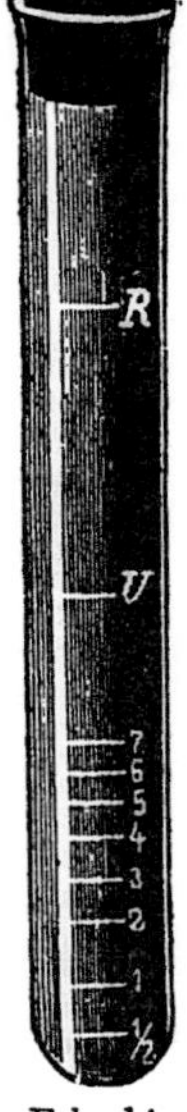

Esbach's Albuminimeter.

Accidental albuminuria is rare and of little importance. We *assume* that the albuminuria is accidental when the filtrate contains large quantities of blood and pus corpuscles and epithelial cells and only a moderate quantity of albumin. In that case the proportionately small amount of albumin is supposed to result from partial solution of the cellular elements.

Chemical determination of albuminuria. For this use freshly voided urine; if not clear, filter.

1. Koch's test. Fill test tube to ¼ its height with urine—if alkaline add a drop of acetic acid—boil and then add 1-10 its volume of dilute nitric acid (sp. gr. 1.18); a permanent precipitate indicates albumin. If a precipitate or turbidity produced by boiling disappears on addition of nitric acid it indicates phosphate of lime.

2. Heller's test. The cold, filtered (and, if necessary, acidulated) urine is carefully poured on concentrated nitric acid, so as to form a layer on the same. If albumin is present a white or cloudy ring is formed in the test tube where the urine comes in contact with the nitric acid.

3. Acetic acid ferro-cyanide of potash test. To the filtered urine add a quantity of acetic acid and then a few drops of a 5% solution of potassium ferrocyanide; the presence of albumin produces a white precipitate.

If the addition of acetic acid produces cloudiness mucin is present; in this case filter the urine. The mucin may also be precipitated with acetate of lead before making the test.

4. A few crystals of salicylsulphonic acid added to a few cubic centimeters of urine will, if albumin is present, produce a cloudy precipitate.

5. The addition of a few grains of trichlor-acetic acid added to clear filtered urine produces a thick turbidity on the bottom of the vessel near the reagent.

6. In case only a limited quantity of urine is obtainable, the following method is recommended: Heat distilled water to boiling point in a test tube, add the urine drop by drop. If albumin is present the drops become turbid in the water, and by continuing the addition of the urine, the water also becomes turbid.

The methods here given suffice for the clinical demonstration of albumin. For a quantitative determination of the albumin preserve the tubes containing the precipitate and thus the sediment, which consists of albumin, may be compared from day to day. For this purpose Esbach's albuminimeter is both simple and practical. See fig. 40. [Similar tubes can be obtained in the United States.] It is used as follows: Fill the tube with urine to the mark U (urine), then add reagents sufficient to fill the tube up to the mark R (reagents) as follows:

citric acid, 2.0 cc,
picro-nitric acid 1.0 cc,
distilled water 100.0 cc;

put on a stopper, shake well, and let stand 24 hours. The sediment which consists of albumin can then be read off in fractions of 1-10%. This instrument gives good results providing the amount of albumin present does not much exceed 0.2%; in that case dilute before testing the urine, say to 50% or 25%, by adding one or three volumes of water respectively; the result must then be multiplied by 2 or 4 according to the dilution.

Albuminuria occurs:

In all febrile diseases, especially in acute infectious diseases; contagious pleuro-pneumonia of the horse and in influenza.

In acute and chronic affections of the kidneys.

In venous congestion, hence in organic heart disease, emphysema and in the various forms of heaves

In blood diseases; leukæmia, anæmia.

In nervous affections, epilepsy, eclampsia.

II. Albumosuria. Examinations for albumoses have only recently become of importance, since simpler methods have been discovered. The occurrence of albumoses depends upon entirely different conditions than those which produce albuminuria. Albumosuria is not caused by inflammation of the kidneys, by disorders of circulation nor by anemia. Changes in the composition of the blood play the chief role here. Albumoses cannot be determined by boiling the fluid containing them, nor by the addition of acids. It is only in the absence of other albuminous substances (albumin, globulin, mucin) and various other pigments that their presence can be determined.

Chemical determination of albumoses. Take 10 cc of unfiltered urine and acidulate with a 20% solution of acetic acid. If the reaction of the urine is acid, two or three drops will suffice, if alkaline, it requires more. Add 5cc of a 20% solution of acetate of lead, boil and filter. Add to the filtrate a solution of caustic potash until precipitates no longer occur; it may require 15cc or more of the potash solution to bring about this result; it is important to use sufficient potash solution as otherwise the reaction will not occur. The filtrate is now subjected to the biuret reaction: Add five or six drops of a solution of sodium hydrate, then add, carefully, one or two, or at the most, three, drops of a 10% solution of sulphate of copper. If albumoses are present a reddish violet color is produced. This test is the simplest and most reliable for testing the urine of animals, since all substances that might otherwise have interfered with the test are removed.

Schulz's method is very simple and reliable. Filter the urine and add several volumnes of alcohol to precipitate all of the albuminous substances. Filter again and treat the residue (precipitate) with a stream of water; this dissolves the albumoses, if present, and then the biuret-reaction is applied to this solution.

Albumoses occur in the urine in the course of abscess formation in the internal organs of the body (Strangles), and as a result of the absorption of extensive exudates in the course of influenza of horses, peritonitis and pleuritis.

The determination of albumoses is of clinical importance for the determination of suspected abscess formation in internal organs.

III. Hemaglobinuria. The fact that urine contains blood may often be recognized by its color alone; light red urine, resembling meat water, (oxyhemoglobin) is rare. As a rule it has a muddy brownish red color (methemoglobin). A diagnosis cannot be based upon the color alone, a chemical and microscopical examination is necessary.

Chemical determination. Add caustic potash or soda until the urine is distinctly alkaline, then boil as in albumin test. This converts the hemoglobin into hematin, it is precipitated with the earthy salts and gives them a reddish brown color.

The difference between oxyhemoglobin and methemoglobin must be determined with the spectroscope. Oxyhemoglobin gives *two* absorption bands between D and E, methemoglobin gives *one* between C and D.

The presence of hemoglobin may be due to admixture of blood as such (*hematuria*) or to hemoglobin alone (hemoglobinuria).

Hematuria is recognized by microscopic examination of the sediment and the detection of blood corpuscles. The admixture of blood can occur in the kidney, the pelvis of the kidney, the bladder or the urethra. It occurs most frequently in red water, acute nephritis, renal calculi, hemorrhagic infarction of the kidney, pyelonephritis, acute cystitis, cystic calculi.

Hemoglobinuria consists in the presence of hemoglobin (without the blood corpuscles) in the urine. The coloring matter is derived either from the blood or the muscles. Accordingly we distinguish:

a. *Hematogenic* or *toxemic hemoglobinuria* in red-water of cattle and in Texas fever, also in bad cases of poisoning which cause decomposition of the red corpuscles, in extensive burns and in the course of severe infectious diseases.

b. *Myogenic* or *rheumatic* hemoglobinuria in azoturia.

c. **Indican** — indoxyl sulphate of potash $C_8 H_6 N K S O_4$, occurs in all urine in moderate amount. It is derived from the *indol* C_8H_7N formed in the alimentary canal during putrefaction of albumin; indol is oxydized into *indoxyl* $C_8H_6N O H$ and then combines with sulphate of potash to form *indoxyl sulphate of potash* — indican. The urine of the horse contains on an average, 184 mg. per liter.

If rapid putrefaction of albuminous substances takes place in the alimentary canal the amount of indican is increased; this is particularly the case in digestive disorders accompanied with diminished peristalsis, digestion and absorption. Constipation of the ileum produces the largest amount of indican; impaction of the colon on the other hand, is attended with much less indican formation.

Diarrhea is attended with diminished indican formation.

Test for Indican. Mix equal parts of urine and pure nitric acid in a test tube, shake well; then add, drop by drop, followed by repeated shaking, a fresh solution of chloride of lime, this causes the formation and precipitation of indigo, recognized by its blue color. The addition of chloroform followed by thorough agitation, dissolves the indigo and the resultant blue solution settles at the bottom of the test tube.

Quantitative Determination, according to Bauer. Take 20 cc of the urine, slightly acidulated with acetic acid, precipitate with two, or if necessary, with four cc of a 20% solution of acetate of lead, filter through a dry filter paper; take 11 or 12 cc (enough to represent 10 cc of urine) of the filtrate and add an equal volume of Obermayer's Reagent (solution of chloride of iron in fuming hydrochloric acid 2:1000). Upon the appearance of a dark coloration, always occurring in urine containing indican in any quantity, allow the solution to stand a few minutes, add 20 cc of chloroform and shake thoroughly for about fifteen seconds. After a short time, when the chloroform has settled to the bottom of the test tube as a clear blue solution, pour a portion of the chloroform into an absorption-test-vessel of 4mm depth, place the vessel upon a piece of paper adjacent to the colors in the table, and by comparison determine which solution has a corresponding amount of indican. If the color corresponds in shade to that given in plate I, the urine contains 50 mg of indigo blue per liter, if it corresponds to the shade indicated in plate II, it contains 100 mg per liter, etc. If the shade is darker than indicated in plate VI, add an equal volume of distilled water, or, if necessary, several volumes; make comparisons as explained and multiply the result with two, three, etc., as the case may be.

d. Bile Pigments. Choleurea. Under normal conditions bile pigments do not occur in the blood of animals and are therefore also absent in the urine. Bile pigments are always formed in the liver; if in the course of disease they are found in the blood (cholemia) or in the urine (choluria) they must have originated in the liver. Bile passes into the blood as a result of the congestion of bile in the larger bile ducts from whence it passes through the lymphatics to the thoracic duct and the general circulation.

Of the bile pigments, bilirubin alone occurs in the Urine containing bile pigments, is usually of a dark color, golden yellow, yellowish brown or greenish yellow and the foam is yellow. The foam of urine free from admixture of bile pigments is white.

Test for bile pigments. For the qualitative determination of bile, we make use of Gmelin's test. Into a test tube containing about three cc of concentrated nitric acid with an admixture of fuming nitric acid (NO2) add a small quantity of the urine to be tested being careful that no mixing of the liquids occurs. (In case the urine has an alkaline reaction it should first be acidulated). If bile pigments are present, various colors will appear at the point of contact of the two liquids, of which the green color alone is characteristic.

This antiquated test of Gmelin has been superseded by newer and better methods. The following are recommended:

Rosenbach's test. Filter the urine through a piece of white filter paper; to the paper thus saturated with the urine add a drop of nitric acid. If bile pigments are present, the characteristic color rings will appear encircling the drop.

According to **Dragendorf,** this test is neatly performed by dropping some of the urine on a porous plate of earthenware and then adding the nitric acid as above.

Ehrlich's test. Add one volume of 30% acetic acid to the urine. Then, drop by drop, add Ehrlich's reagent (1 gram acid sulfanil in aqueous solution, 15cc. HCl, and 0.1 gram Sodium Nitrite, water sufficient to make 1,000 grams. If Bilirubin is present the mass gets dark. If much glacial acetic acid is added or if boiled, the fluid becomes intensely violet in color. Hydrochloric acid may be substituted for the glacial acetic acid—producing a beautiful violet red.

Schmidt's test. Very valuable for dark colored urine or blood serum. Add Sodium bicarbonate until reaction is alkaline. Add 10% solution of Barium chloride until precipitates cease. If bilirubin is present the precipitate is yellow, otherwise white. Centrifuge the precipitate, wash with water, mix with alcohol containing 5% hydrochloric acid by volume. If bilirubin is present, the supernatant fluid, especially if heated, is bluish green. If the fluid becomes brown add a few drops of hydrogen peroxide to complete oxydation whereupon the brown color becomes green.

Choleuria occurs: In retention of bile in the liver as a result of occlusion of the ductus choledochus in duodenal catarrh, presence of tumors, parasites, concrements.

In lupinosis and phosphorus poisoning as a result of swelling of the liver and obstruction of the bile ducts.

In all of these cases the feces are deficient in normal bile contents and as a result appear of a lighter color.

When the bile secreted is of abnormal consistency (hypercholia), its flow is interrupted and stagnation occurs. This results in the course of the destruction of large numbers of red blood corpuscles; also in the course of haemoglobinaemia, lumbago, septicemia, pyemia, burns, internal hemorrhage, prolonged chloroform narcosis and similar poisonings. In addition to choleuria the feces also contain much bile.

e. **Grape sugar, Glycosuria,** by means ordinarily employed can be detected in urine in disease only, viz. in diabetes mellitus. In horses this disease has been observed in a few instances only, in dogs it is common. We suspect the presence of sugar in polyuria when the specific gravity of the urine is high.

Fig. 41.

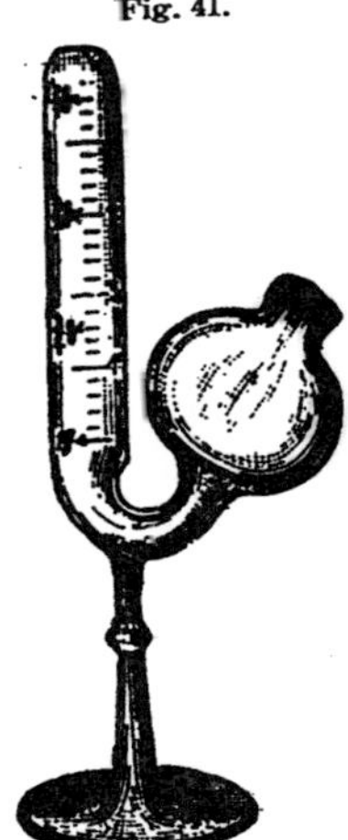

Fermentation tube.

Chemical determination. If albumin is present this must first be removed by adding acetic acid, boiling, and filtering. Then add to 10 cc urine 1 cc caustic potash solution; if this produces cloudiness, filter again. Then add about 3 drops of a 10% solution of sulphate of copper. The appearance of a light blue color is in itself an indication of grape sugar; now heat the fluid, if grape sugar is present an orange yellow precipitate which gradually extends downward is formed at the surface; this is an oxide of copper.

This test (Trommer's test) is by no means reliable for horse urine because the latter contains other bodies that have a reducing power: *Pyrocatechin,* etc. On the other hand, substances that prevent the reduction (or precipitation) of oxide of copper may be present. Pure grape sugar, when added to horse urine, can sometimes not be detected at all by means of Trommer's test. In all cases of doubt we must therefore resort to the fermentation test, as follows:

Boil 20 cc of urine that has been freed from albumin, let cool and add a piece of baker's yeast as large as a pea, shake thoroughly, pour into a fermentation tube and close the latter with metallic mercury. Keep the tube at room temperature for 24-48 hours. If sugar is present fermentation will set in and the CO_2 thus produced will collect in the top of the tube where the percentage is indicated by a graduated scale.

$$C_6 H_{12} O_6 = 2C_2 H_5 OH_2 + C O_2$$

Grape sugar = alcohol + carbondioxide.

This test can of course be relied upon only when we

are assured of the quality of the yeast and that it is free from traces of sugar.

The **phenylhydrazin test** ($C_6H_8N_2$) of V. Jacksch (Modification of Esch'baum) is very reliable for the urine of the dog (Regenbogen). Mix 5 drops of phenylhydrazin, 20 drops of glacial acetic acid and 50 drops of urine in a test tube and boil gently for one minute; add 25 drops of officinal sodium hydrate solution and again raise to boiling point. Allow the mixture to settle for 12-24 hours and then make a microscopic examination of the sediment. If the urine contained sugar bunches of yellow, needle-like crystals of phenylglukosazone will be found.

Fig. 42.

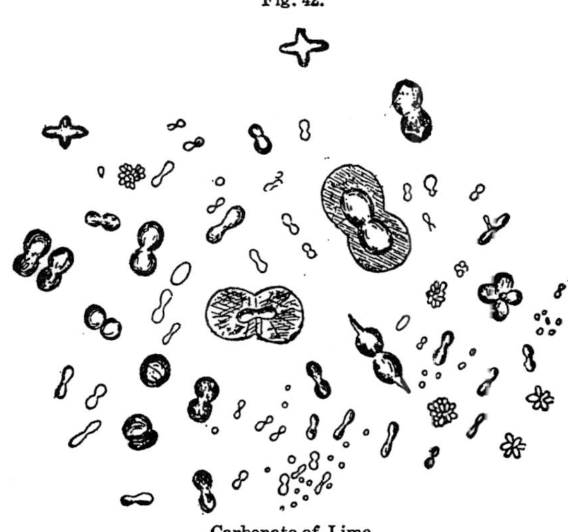

Carbonate of Lime.

Lactose occurs in the urine of cows advanced in pregnancy, disappears after calving and reappears when the milk ducts become obstructed.

C. Microscopical Examination of the Urine.

If the examination thus far conducted reveals any important alterations, we complete the same with the microscope. A microscopic examination of the urine in diseases of the urinary organs is of even greater importance than a chemical analysis.

Method. Pour some of the urine into a conical glass, previously stirring the same with a glass rod to be sure to get an average sample. The urine is then set away to allow the solid particles to settle out; with horse urine this is a rather slow process. To prevent decomposition during the process of sedimentation, add a few drops of chloroform. Remove some of the sediment with a pipette and examine a drop on a slide, under the microscope.

A. Crystalline Constituents of Urine.

The reaction of the urine itself gives us a certain clue as to the character of the sediments. The normal alkaline urine of herbivora contains (see p. 151) carbonate of lime and small quantities of neutral phosphates $Ca_3(PO_4)_2$. Such sediment does not dissolve when heat is applied, but the addition of hydrochloric acid produces solution, and development of CO_2. The sediment which forms in the acid urine of carnivora consists of acid urates and acid phosphates which dissolve on being heated.

To determine accurately the nature of the crystalline sediment a microscopical examination must be made; the forms of the crystals indicate their nature. Amorphous salts can be recognized by micro-chemical tests only.

a. Carbonate of lime crystallizes in globules with radiate markings, if the globules are large a concentric marking

Fig. 43.

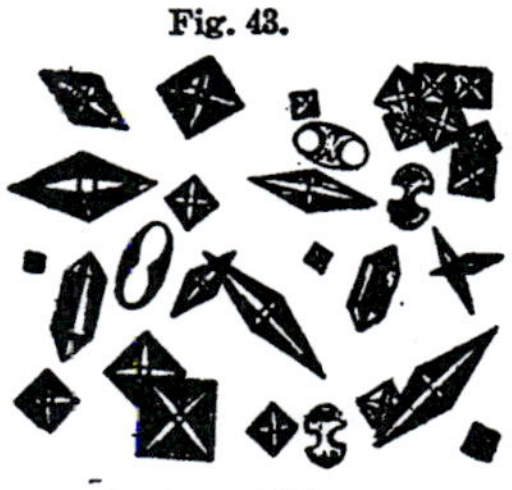

Oxalate of Lime.

Fig. 44.

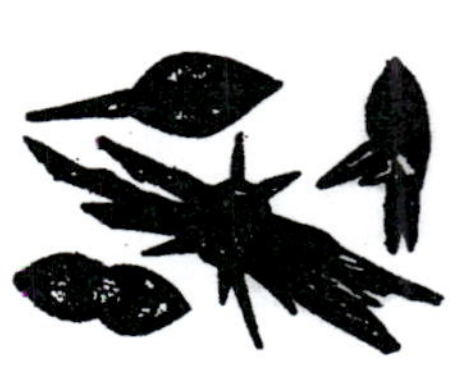

Uric Acid.

can also be observed. Carbonate of lime crystals also occur in form of breakfast rolls, dumb-bells, whetstones and crosses. Amorphous powder of carbonate of lime can be recognized by the fact that the addition of acetic acid causes an evolution of gas.

b. **Oxalate of lime** crystallizes in square octahedra that have strong light-refracting power, other forms occur but are not characteristic. Acetic acid does not affect oxalate of lime, hydrochloric acid dissolves it. It occurs in small quantities in alkaline urine, to a greater extent in acid urine, but is of no importance for diagnostic purposes.

c. **Uric acid and its salts** are normal constituents of the urine of carnivora but traces of them also occur in the urine of herbivora.

They commonly occur as an amorphous powder or in the form of crystals; whetstone, rhombic plates, pointed crys-

Fig. 45.

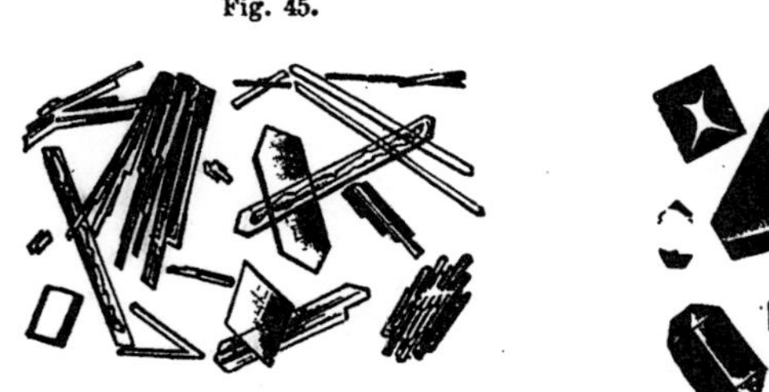

Hippuric Acid.

Fig. 46.

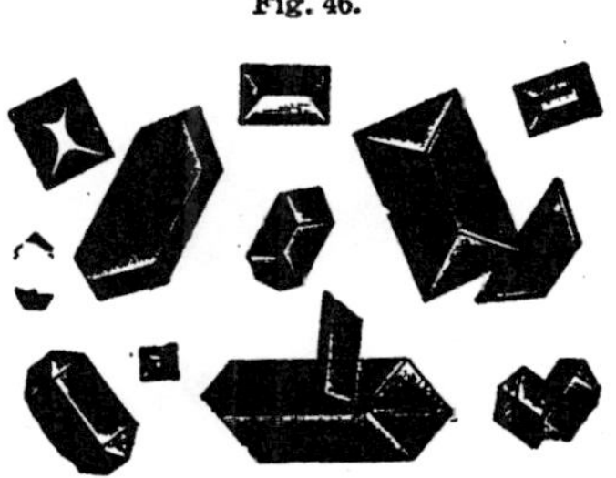

Triplephosphate Crystals.

tals, frequently occurring in the form of minute druses. A characteristic consists in the peculiarity that, on crystallizing, they attract the pigment of the urine which gives them a yellowish brown color. They dissolve in a solution of caustic potash, and they are precipitated in the form of rhombic prisms by the addition of hydrochloric acid.

d. **Hippuric acid** and its salts form rhombic quadrilateral prisms and needles which dissolve in hydrochloric acid Normal constituent of urine of horses.

e. **Triple phosphate of ammonia and magnesia** PO_4MgNH_4 crystallizes in coffin-lid forms, dissolves in acetic acid without giving off gas. Does not occur normally in freshly voided urine, but always forms when urine is exposed to the air for some time (*fermentation*). If found in fresh urine it indicates that ammoniacal fermentation has taken place in the bladder, *cystitis, pyelitis.*

f. **Sulphate of lime,** gypsum, occurs occasionally and in small quantity in the form of columnar prisms or plates in acid urine. It is *abundant* after internal administration of sulphates (Glauber salts). Of no importance.

B. Organized Elements of Urine.

In the diagnosis of diseases of the urinary organs these are of the greatest importance. The addition of Lugol's Solution to the sediment is an aid in recognizing the cellular elements under the microscope.

Fig. 47.

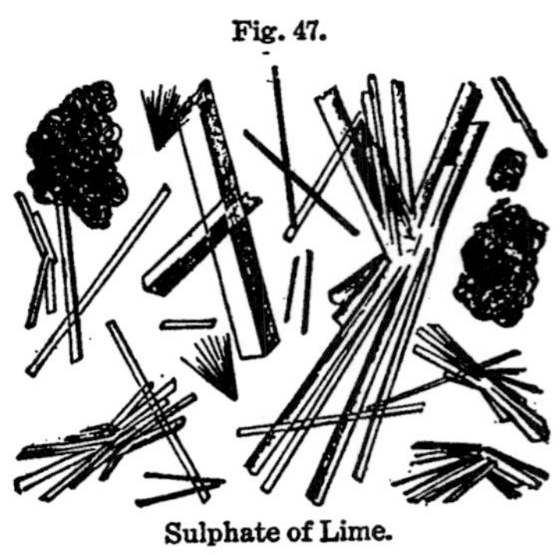

Sulphate of Lime.

g. **Epithelial cells** in small number are found in normal urine, occasionally we find two or three pavement epithelial cells in one cover-glass preparation. On the other hand the finding of epithelial cells from the uriniferous tubules (renal epithelia) is an exception under these conditions. Marked increase of epithelial cells is due to a pathological desquamation, hence is observed in catarrhs and inflammation of the membranes concerned. It is important to be able to recognize the origin of the cells by their form.

Renal epithelium is roundish or more or less cubical and granulated with proportionately large granules and is much smaller than the pavement epithelium of the pelvis of the kidney, the urethra and the bladder. They occur singly or several united and not infrequently show signs of fatty degeneration. Their occurrence indicates a renal affection, *but* whether or not inflammation exists must be determined by further examination of the urine.

Pavement epithelia from the pelvis of the kidney, the urethra and the bladder resemble each other and cannot be distinguished as to their particular source. They are large, flat, polygonal, transparent, nucleated pavement cells. Those coming from the surface layers of the mucous membrane are more roundish or polygonal, those from the deeper layers are more oval, or cone shaped and may contain one or more protoplasmic projections that give them a *toothed* appearance. If a considerable number of such cells are present a catarrhal condition of the corresponding mucous membranes is indicated.

h. **White blood corpuscles** or pus cocci are spherical, granulated, nucleated cells that are *cleared* or become transparent when treated with acetic acid. They may have come from the kidneys or from the urinary tract; if from the kidneys we also find casts, if they occur simultaneously with numerous pavement epithelia and crystals of triplephosphate they come from the bladder.

i. **Red blood corpuscles,** when found in the urine, have lost most of their coloring matter, are pale and swollen. Those coming from the upper portions of the urinary tract have undergone these changes to a greater extent than those coming from the lower portions. Thorough admixture of red corpuscles with the urine, thus retarding sedimentation of the former, points to renal hemorrhage; blood casts always point to renal hemorrhage. Large masses or clots of blood, not thoroughly mixed with the urine, come from the bladder. An admixture of blood with the urine (hematuria) occurs in:

1. Diseases of the kidneys: injuries, hemorrhagic nephritis, embolic nephritis;

2. Diseases of the urinary tract: pyelonephritis, cystitis, red water of cattle, cystic calculi, cystic tumors, injuries of the urethra.

k. **Urinary casts** are cylindrical bodies that were molded in the lumen of the uriniferous tubules. In the urine of the horse we find similar structures under normal conditions; they consist of strings of mucus of variable thickness, sometimes macroscopically visible and granulated with deposits of amorphous carbonate of lime. Addition of acetic acid causes the granules to disappear with the formation of CO_2. In acid urine we find uric acid salts instead. These so called *granule casts, lime casts,* or *cylinderoids* have nothing whatever in common with true urinary casts. They are especially common in the transition stage from oliguria to polyuria.

The true urinary casts are distinguished as follows:

1. *Hyaline casts,* slender, transparent, homogeneous bodies of various sizes and not sharply defined contour. They are rare, occur in health as well as in disease, are of no diagnostic importance and their origin is unknown.

Fig. 48.

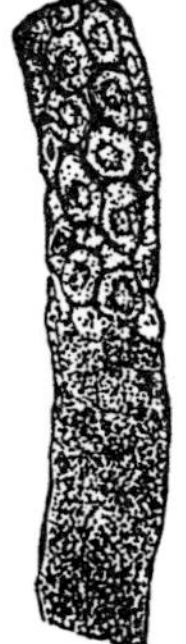

Epithelial Casts.

2. *Epithelial casts* consist of renal epithelia agglutinated with exudates and forced out of the tubules by the pressure of the urine above them. Frequently red and white blood corpuscles are associated with them. Such cylinders, providing they occur in any appreciable numbers, always indicate inflammation of the kidneys. These epithelial cells may also have undergone fatty degeneration. If they contain no cells they are called *granular casts*, and have the same significance as the epithelial cylinders.

Fig. 49.

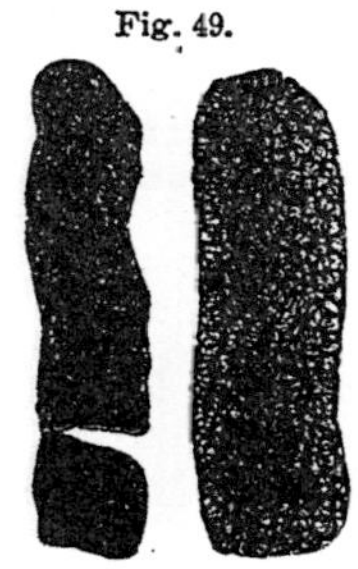

Granular Casts.

3. *Blood corpuscle casts* are formed of agglutinated red corpuscles and are due to renal hemorrhage. If these casts contain many white corpuscles they indicate purulent inflammation (*pus-casts*).

1. **Examination for micro-organisms** is of value in case of fresh urine only, because urine that has been standing for some time will soon become filled with great masses of bacteria and mold fungi from the air. Large numbers of bacteria in *fresh urine* occur in pyelonephritis bacteritica and in chronic cystitis.

Bacillus pyelonephritis bovis will stain according to Gram's method. A cover glass preparation is made from the sediment of the urine, stained with gentian violet, rinsed with water, a few drops of Lugol's solution (Iod. 8, Pot. Iod. 4, Aqua 100) added, then decolorized in alcohol. All bacteria that stain according to Gram's method have now assumed a deep blue color; while all the rest are decolorized. Bac. pyeloneph. appears as a rod with rounded ends, 2-3u long and 0.7u in diameter, evenly stained and usually occurring in little groups.

III. Examination of the Urinary Organs.

Topography. In the horse and cow the left kidney only is accessible for palpation from the rectum, the right kidney lies further forward and cannot be reached by the hand. In the horse the left kidney extends back to about four inches behind the last rib and its inner border is separated from the median line by about the same distance. In the ox it is loosely suspended below the lateral processes of the first lumber vertebrae. Sometimes it may be shifted over to the right side. In the dog the kidneys lie in the lumbar region, the right somewhat more anterior than the left; hence the left kidney can be more easily felt from the outside than the right kidney.

In palpating the kidneys follow the general rules for this method of examination (see p. 23). In pyelonephritis of the ox the kidneys are enlarged and firm, the ureters distended and their walls thickened and firm.

Examination of the bladder, per rectum, in the horse and ox, is quite practicable; in the dog the examination must be made by external palpation. The extent to which the bladder is filled is of importance; if empty, in the horse and cow, it represents a soft pearshaped body lying on the floor of the pelvis. If well filled it can be felt as a distended body projecting far beyond the anterior border of the pelvis. To feel it the hand need not be inserted much further than to the wrist. The contents of the bladder can be removed by a steady but moderate pressure applied with the hand, or by means of the catheter; this may be important to determine whether evacuation is possible. If the bladder is ruptured, which is most common in oxen with urethral calculi, it is permanently small and flabby.

Cystic calculi and tumors in the bladder can be recognized with certainty only when this organ contains little or no fluid contents.

Examination of the urethra is of consequence in male animals, particularly in oxen, when the presence of calculi may be suspected. As a rule these are lodged in the upper or lower portion of the S shaped curve. Pressure exerted at the point where the obstruction is located produces pain. As long as the bladder is not ruptured urine may dribble from the distended urethra. Unfortunately catheterization is impossible in the ox (sharp curves and narrow lumen of urethra) ; in the horse and dog this examination is easy and reliable.

Diseases of the Urinary Apparatus.

Passive hyperaemia of the kidneys occurs as a result of chronic heart and lung troubles. Urine is decreased, sp. gr. increased, albumin present. Symptoms more conspicuous after exertions.

Acute diffuse nephritis. This is primary only in cases of poisoning with irritating substances, otherwise it is a symptom of severe infections. Dysuria, stranguria, pain in the region of the kidneys, stiff gait and crooked back. Considerable diminution of renal secretion (anuria), thick and viscid, turbid, high sp. gr., acid, much albumin. Microscopic examination most important: granular casts, renal epithelia and blood corpuscles. Stupefaction, difficult breathing, oedematous swellings.

Nephritis suppurativa. Secondary affection and usually of less importance than the primary disease. Intermittent fever, exhaustion, emaciation, urine contains albumin, pus corpuscles and microorganisms.

Chronic nephritis. No fever, develops very slowly. Anorexia, exhaustion, emaciation. Pulse strong and hard, heart hypertrophied. Increased amount of urine, low sp. gr., amount of albumin slight, few epithelial cells and casts.

Cystitis, inflammation of the bladder. Continuous efforts to urinate, hence small quantities or only a few drops are voided at a time. Urination painful, restlessness, groaning, animals remain for a long time in a "urinating attitude." Urine cloudy, alkaline, slimy or purulent sediment, ammoniacal odor. Pus corpuscles, red blood corpuscles, numerous pavement epithelia, phosphate of ammonia and magnesia.

Retentio urinae. Retention of urine. Complete (ischuria) or partial suppression of urination; in the latter case it is voided in drops and with symptoms of pain. Palpation of the bladder very important: distention, pain on pressure. Animals indisposed, inactive, do not lie down, appetite diminished, pulse increased, sweating. After rupture of bladder has occurred the pains disappear, animals feel more at ease, bladder is empty. Then come chills, high fever, urinous odor of transpired air.

Incontinentia urinae. Paralysis of bladder. Involuntary flow of urine, especially during motion.

Hematuria is a chronic productive cystitis of the ox, with tendency to hemorrhage. Blood corpuscles and clots in the urine.

Hemoglobinuria of the ox. Hemoglobinemia. Fever, partial loss of appetite, diarrhea. Urine light red to dark red, foams readily, urination painful, reaction at first acid, later on alkaline, contains hemoglobin, on boiling coagulates as gelatinous mass.

Pyelonephritis bacteritica boum. This is a chronic purulent inflammation of the ureters and pelvis of the kidneys which spreads to the kidneys and is caused by a specific bacillus. Gradual emaciation and general depression. Intermittent fever. Urine thick and slimy, cloudy, gray or grayish brown, white and red blood corpuscles, casts, numerous pavement epithelia, crystals of triple phosphate, and bacilli, Bacillus pyelonephritidis boum. Stain according to Gram, 2-3 micra long, 0.6-0.7 micra in diameter, non-motile, straight or slightly bent, rounded at the ends.

Urolithiasis, stones, concretions and sediments (gravel) cause catarrhal inflammation and periodical hemorrhages. Urethral concrements produce retention of urine.

Diseases of Tissue Metabolism.

Diabetes insipidus, polyuria, pissing, is an independent disease in which large quantities of clear watery urine are passed continuously. Daily quantity of urine passed equaling as high as 30 liters. Urine as clear as water or slightly yellow, acid, sp. gr. 1001-1010, no albumin, little indican. Diminished appetite, desire for alkalies, [earth, etc.] emaciation.

Diabetes mellitus, sugar in the urine, is very rare in horses, more common in dogs. Polyuria, ravenous appetite and thirst, rapid emaciation. Urine has high sp. gr., 1024-1045, and contains grape sugar.

10. The Sexual Apparatus.

Most of the organs of the sexual apparatus may, for the greater part, be subjected to direct inspection and palpation; their examination should be conducted according to general rules, care being observed that no parts are overlooked. For evident reasons the female sexual organs are more frequently affected with diseases than those of the male. Most of these diseases belong to the field of obstetrics.

I. Abnormally increased sexual desire manifests itself not only by sexual excitement but also by psychic disturbances and altered sensibility, these often resembling diseases of the central nervous system. In females this condition is known as *nymphomania,* in males as *satyriasis;* continued erections of the penis is called *priapism.*

Mares are usually very ticklish and easily excited, if touched with the hand or harness they squeak or cry out, switch their tail, back up against persons or against the wagon tongue, kick, urinate, and can be used for their regular work only when special care is exercised. In rare cases they may act like dummies (general depression of the sensorium) and show symptoms of hyperesthesia.

Cows show symptoms of great restlessness, are very excitable, bellow frequently, attack strangers, etc. Milk secretion is reduced, the milk has a bad taste and sometimes curdles when boiled.

In horses and bulls satyriasis manifests itself by restlessness and excitable, sometimes vicious, actions.

In many cases the cause of these conditions cannot be ascertained; in cows tuberculosis of the ovaries, in horses cryptorchism, is often the cause.

II. The vulva. In bitches we observe swelling of the vulva and a bloody mucous discharge at the oestral period. In cows a tough glassy mucus is discharged just before parturition. This mucus comes from the neck of the uterus which it served to close.

A slight swelling of the vulva occurs in vesicular eruption of this region; small vesicles the size of a millet seed, and swelling may also occur in the adjacent skin in this condition. In puerperal septicemia the vulva swells conspicuously.

In torsion of the uterus the vulva is retracted and drawn into folds; however, exploration per vagina is necessary to definitely determine this condition.

Discharge from the inferior commissure of the vulva and soiling of the surrounding skin and tail are observed in:

a. Catarrh of the vagina and uterus. In chronic catarrh (fluor albus) the discharge is of a thick slimy character and glassy; in acute catarrh the discharge is of a thin slimy character and discolored.

b. Retention of the afterbirth; an ill-smelling, discolored fluid mixed with fragments of the fetal membranes is discharged.

c. Vesicular eruption; the discharge is slight, slimy or purulent, sometimes mixed with blood.

d. Tuberculosis; slight, chronic, muco-purulent discharge containing tubercle bacilli.

Relaxation of the broad ligaments occurs not only immediately before parturition but also in the course of ovarian diseases (cysts) and diseases of the uterus and its neck.

III. Vaginal mucous membrane. Whenever there is discharge from the vagina the vaginal mucous membrane should be examined.

Method. Grasp the tail near its root, raise it well up, and let it rest on the back of the other hand, thus leaving the fingers of that hand free to open the lips of the vulva. In order to examine deeper-lying parts an assistant should hold the tail and the operator can then insert his whole hand, which must be previously covered with oil. After thorough palpation in this manner the other hand may also be inserted, the vaginal walls spread apart, and their mucous membrane inspected; here artificial light may be of advantage. A vaginal speculum is not absolutely necessary for these examinations.

By means of direct examinations like these, affections of the vagina can best be observed and their character determined. In vesicular eruption yellowish gray nodules, vesicles or ulcers, the size of a millet seed, are found on the slightly and diffusely reddened mucous membrane. After healing, light specks that indicate the position of former vesicles and ulcers can be observed for some time.

In torsion of the uterus the vagina is contracted, and the mucous membrane is drawn into twisted folds. The examination of the uterus and the explanation of changes in that organ belong to the field of obstetrics.

IV. The udder. In the examination of cows the udder must never be neglected. Inquire at least as to quantity and quality of the milk. Observe the color of the skin and note any changes that may have taken place. The teats of cows and sheep may be affected with pox, in foot and mouth disease the teats of cows may be covered with blisters; we also find milk fistulae. Observe also the relative size of the different quarters of the udder and the condition of the surface; note the size, position, and direction of the teats. In palpation each quarter should be separately felt, its size and consistency noted and sensitive or knotted areas observed. The teats should be soft and the milk canal should not be felt; if thickenings or swellings exist, their location, extent, size and form should be determined. Finally, milk every teat in order to determine the ease with which the fluid can be drawn, notice the size of the stream and the character of the milk, whether it is clotted or bloody: A microscopical examination of abnormal milk is not necessary but may be of value in some cases. To determine whether a cow is "fresh" a microscopical examination of the milk for the colostrum bodies or corpuscles must be made.

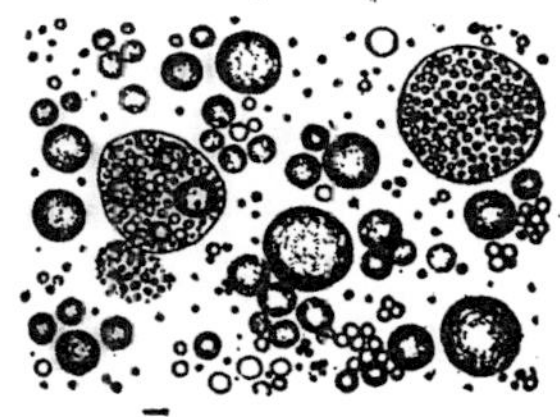

Fig. 50. Colostral Milk.

Harpooning the udder according to Ostertag. The operation may be performed on the standing animal, but better results can be obtained if the animal is cast and secured.

Wash the field of operation with soap and water, rinse with 2 per cent. lysol solution, following this with 50 per cent. alcohol. With hooked forceps grasp the skin overlying the suspicious area in the udder and at the fold thus produced incise the skin and underlying facia with scissors, grasp the tissues with the thumb and index finger of the left hand and insert the harpoon with the right. When the suspected tissue has been reached give the harpoon a half turn and withdraw it quickly. The cutaneous wound is closed with artery forceps which are allowed to remain ten minutes, whereupon the wound is sealed with iodoformcollodion.

Cows thus treated will give bloody milk for a few days, but if carefully performed the operation is not dangerous.

Tubercles, if contained in tissue thus removed, can usually be recognized with the aid of a simple lens. If the examination gives negative results it is advisable to repeat the operation. Tubercle bacilli can always be demonstrated in the tubercles.

In this method a positive diagnosis alone is of any value. We can not rely upon negative results. This method is of value in cases of suspected tuberculosis where we fail to get a tuberculin reaction, or when a suspected quarter is dry and the possiblity of a direct examination of the milk is excluded.

Bacteriological Diagnosis of Udder Tuberculosis According to Ostertag.

The most reliable means of recognizing tuberculosis of the udder consists in the inoculation of Guinea pigs with a sample of milk from the suspected udder.

To obtain reliable results the milk must be procured with proper precautions: Wash the udder with warm water until it is clean, follow this with 50 per cent alcohol and then dry with absorbent cotton. Discard the first ten cc of milk drawn.

One cc of whole milk is used for the inoculation. Inject this into the muscles of the inner posterior region of the thigh. Upon the appearance of firm, hard, painless and well defined nodules the size of small peas or larger, representing the lymph glands near the point of inoculation, the animals may be killed. These nodules may appear as early as the tenth day after inoculation. If the nodules do not make their appearance, the Guniea pigs are killed at the end of six weeks. The presence of tubercle bacilli in the lymphatic glands or in the internal organs demonstrates the existense of tuberculosis.

V. Diseases of the male sexual organs are usually of a surgical nature. In vesicular eruption we find vesicles, pustules and ulcers, or scars, on the penis. To examine stallions or bulls they may be led up to a mare (or cow) which usually results in a voluntary protrusion of the organ. In bulls manipulation with the hand may answer the same purpose In glanders the testicles may reveal the presence of tumors

Diseases of the Sexual Organs.

Torsio uteri, torsion of the womb, of interest in internal medicine only when parturition or pregnancy is excluded. Animals are restless, kick belly with hind feet and have pains of labor. Examination of vagina gives necessary information.

Vaginitis (colpitis), inflammation of vagina. Symptoms vary much, according to degree and character of the affection. If inflammation is severe, general health is affected. Animals make frequent attempts to urinate; small quantities of urine passed at a time; animals remain long in a "urinating attitude." Examination of vagina gives necessary information.

Endometritis, inflammation of the womb. Follows parturition; intensity of disease varies. General health more or less disturbed, fever, discharge from vagina which varies according to character of inflammation, is observed particularly when animals lie down. Soiled tail, examination of womb according to general rules of obstetrics is always indicated.

Tuberculosis of the Uterus and the Vagina. Animals in oestrum but no conception. Vulva asymmetrically enlarged or retracted. Often muco-purulent discharge. Nodules or ulcers, size of millet seed, on mucous membrane. Orificium uteri usually relaxed. Uterus enlarged, diffuse or nodular. Fallopian tubes tortuous unyielding strands, nodulated.

Mastitis, inflammation of udder, garget.

1. Mastitis interstitialis. Fever and hot, rather firm and painful swelling of udder. Quantity of milk decreased, quality not affected.

2. Mastitis catarrhalis. Udder evenly enlarged, soft and elastic, hot. Teats swollen, hot, sometimes reddened. Milk resembling whey. Fever, loss of appetite. Infectious catarrhal mastitis is a special form of catarrhal mastitis, infectious, milk yellowish. Usually all four quarters affected.

3. Mastitis parenchymatosa. As a rule only one quarter affected. Fever, appetite diminished, rumination interrupted, constipation. One-quarter of the udder enlarged, firm, hot, sensitive. The teat of the affected udder is usually free from inflammatory symptoms, the milk secretion is greatly decreased, yellowish, contains muco-purulent flakes which usually contain numerous streptococci.

4. Mastitis tuberculosa. A few nodular enlargements, otherwise the udder is tough and flabby. Supramammary glands enlarged. Tubercle bacilli in milk.

Vesicular eruption [coital exanthema] is an acute infectious vesicular exanthema of the mucous membrane of the vagina and the penis. Period of incubation 3-6 days. The vesicles develop into little ulcers.

Mal du coit [seen in U. S. in imported stallions]. Period of incubation 8 days to 2 months. Swelling of the vulva and penis, formation of vesicles and ulcers. Frequent attempts to urinate, increased sexual desire, urticariform, swellings of skin, paralysis of hind parts.

Infectious Catarrhal Vaginitis. A chronic catarrh of the vaginal mucous membrane, frequently extending to the uterus. Very contagious. Incubation period 2-3 days. General health not affected. At first swelling and tenderness of the vulva, frequent urination. Visible mucous membrane of vagina yellowish red, covered with muco-purulent mass. One or two days later, numerous milliform, dark red, firm nodules in the region of the clittoris. Later these become pale and transparent. In bulls, simple catarrh without nodules. In cows vesicles, pustules or ulcers never occur.

II. The Nervous System.

Diseases of the central nervous system can be recognized only by the disturbed function of its parts, a physical examination of the diseased parts is out of the question. We must therefore subject each function to a careful examination and draw conclusions as to the parts affected from the character of the disturbed physiological processes and conditions. To diagnose diseases of the central nervous system requires a knowledge of the location of the principal functions.

Preliminary remarks on anatomy and physiology. All efferent (motor) psychic (conscious and volitional) fibres **originate in** the *cortex of the cerebrum*, and all sensory fibres and fibres of special sense that conduct perceptible impulses **terminate** in the *cortex of the cerebrum.* The voluntary motor fibres (psycho-motor or cortico-muscular tracts, or simply pyramidal tracts) course from the cortex, through the pons Varolii to the anterior pyramids of the medulla oblongata. Here most of these fibres cross over to the opposite side (motor decussation) and go to the motor nerves of the extremities, through the lateral columns of the spinal cord. A few fibres that do not decussate as above described course along the anterior columns of the spinal cord and gradually pass over to the other side like the rest, but through the white commissure along the course of the cord.

Hence destructive processes in one hemisphere result in motor and sensory paralysis on the opposite side of the body.

The cerebral hemispheres are also the seat of all psychical activities; they are the seat of thought, volition and sensation. Many motor centers are also found in the cerebral cortex and hence inflammatory conditions of this region may be attended with convulsive movements of the muscles.

The midbrain (crura cerebri, corpora quadrigemini and optic thalami) is the seat of the entire mechanism, harmony and equilibrium of all motions. Animals with both hemispheres removed, but with the midbrain intact can retain their equilibrium under the most varied conditions. Inflammatory irritation of the midbrain produces involuntary movements.

The cerebellum harmonizes or co-ordinates the movements of the body by regulating the succession of muscular contractions.

The spinal cord, besides conducting impulses to and from the brain, contains reflex centers which, when stimulated by afferent impulses, cause certain kinds of important movements (defense, flight, etc). These movements are carried out independent of any action on part of the brain, as is easily proved on decapitated animals or where the spinal cord has been cut through. The thus isolated cord is as prompt as ever in producing reflex actions. The lumbar cord is the special center for defecation and urination, which also depend on reflex activity.

To be able to recognize normal conditions as well as to determine the presence and seat of pathological changes in the central nervous system, observe the following points:

I. Psychic Functions.
II. Sensibility.
III. Motility.

I. Psychic Functions.

Since the cerebrum and particularly its cortex is the seat of all psychic activities, disease of the same must interfere with normal *thought, feeling,* and *volition;* movements, sensations and perceptions of peripheral parts occur unconsciously. The general mechanism, harmony and equilibrium of muscular movements may be entirely intact in this condition. Mental disturbances occur in a great many infectious diseases, in febrile diseases in general, in the course of intoxications (poisonings) of varied kinds, and in local diseases of the brain itself.

Therefore, mental disturbances can be ascribed to local causes only when the possibility of a general cause is eliminated. The disturbances in question consist of abnormal *excitability* or of abnormal *depression.*

Mental excitement is the result of cerebral irritation — as observed in acute cerebritis. Horses become restless, neigh, refuse to be led, try to tear loose from the halter, step to and fro, paw, climb up into the manger, are anxious and easily frightened. Cattle bellow, snort, shake their heads, jump around, and into the manger. Dogs manifest their restlessness by an aimless running about, barking, howling and even biting. Pigs squeal, crawl under the litter, run about, climb over obstacles and jump up against walls. Similar symptoms are also observed in rabies, acute tubercular meningitis, malignant catarrhal fever of the ox and in anthrax.

Symptoms of mental depression frequently follow those of excitement. The animals droop the head, rest it on the crib or feeding rack, eyes half closed, take no interest in their surroundings, do not recognize familiar persons, run against obstacles, etc. In feeding they grab the food with the incisor teeth, chew slowly and "languidly," stop without a motive when food is still in the mouth and between the lips. In drinking they plunge their mouth into the water and often "chew" it. It is hard to make them move, they step around clumsily, won't "get over" when commanded to

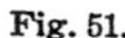

Fig. 51.

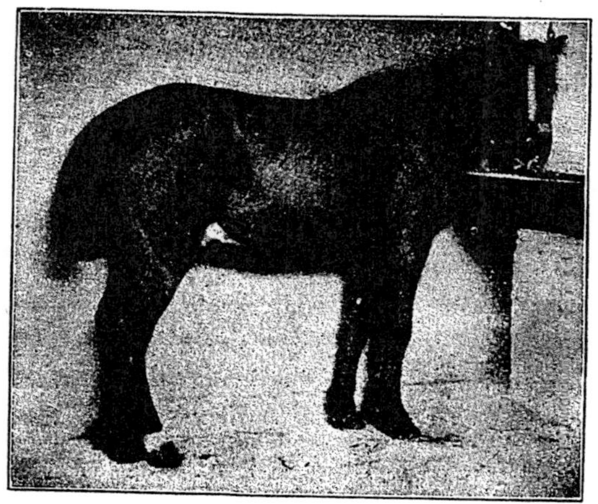

Horse with chronic hydrocephalus.

do so; they are hard to guide when driven, try to stay over on one side; if badly affected they cannot be used for service because they do not recognize commands. According to the degree of mental depression we recognize:

Dullness;

Somnolency, sleepiness, drowsiness, from which the patient is easily roused.

Sopor, profound sleep, rousing difficult.

Coma, complete insensibility.

A dulling of the psychic functions occurs in;

1. All acute infectious diseases; contagious pleuropneumonia, influenza, Rinderpest, anthrax, horse, distemper, dog distemper, septicemia, Rothlauf of swine, etc.

2. All severe febrile diseases.

3. Chronic affections of the brain: blind staggers, turnsick of sheep, second stage of acute cerebritis and cerebral hyperemia.

4. Poisoning with narcotics.

5. Icterus, uraemia.

6. Chronic gastric and intestinal affections of the horse.

Dizziness (vertigo) and **syncope (fainting)** are suddenly occurring temporary disturbances of consciousness and loss of equilibrium. Animals suddenly become unsteady in gait or standing position, sway, reel, stagger and sometimes fall to the ground. The cause may consist of the presence of parasites in the brain, hemorrhages, tumors, abscesses, *passive* cerebral hyperemia (compression of jugulars by harness), aortic insufficiency or stenosis, also the action of glaring light ("ocular vertigo"), irritations of the external auditory meatus, and of the nasal mucous membrane by parasites, finally also of poisoning with certain plants.

II. Sensibility.

The sensibility is tested by artificial stimulation, sticking a finger into the ear, flipping the nose with the finger, stepping on the coronet, pin pricks. In testing the general sensibility observe that no inflammatory condition exists in the part "tested." Peripheral irritation may give rise to spinal reflex actions, e. g. the hoof may be raised without any consciousness of the act on part of the animal either as to the act or stimulus producing it. For this reason the general behavior of the whole animal must be taken into account in testing its sensibility. If dogs cry out during such an examination, or test we may conclude that conscious feeling exists.

Decreased sensibility is called *hypesthesia,* absence of sensibility is called *anesthesia,* abnormally increased sensibility is called *hyperesthesia.* Sometimes sensibility is *retarded;* this is indicated when the reaction occurs an unusually long time after the stimulus is applied.

Hyperesthesia is most frequently seen in old ticklish mares, also in lumbar prurigo of sheep and in the first stages of cerebritis.

Diminished sensibility is observed in chronic affections of the brain, immobility, tumors, second stage of acute cerebritis, parturient fever, second stage of cerebro-spinal meningitis, and in narcotic poisonings.

III. Motility.

In morbid conditions affecting the cerebral hemispheres only we observe no serious disturbances in motility because the mid brain and the cerebellum are the seat of co-ordinated movements.

a. **Spasms,** or cramps, are involuntary muscular contractions. Spasms of short duration, alternating with relaxations, are called *clonic spasms;* if they are very slight, uniform, rapid, and locally limited we call it *trembling;* if they affect large areas or extend over the whole body we call them *convulsions.* Clonic spasms are observed in partial and general epilepsy and in inflammatory affections of the brain and spinal cord (common after dog distemper). *Tonic* or *tetanic* spasms are muscular contractions that continue for some time without relaxation. They are characteristic for tetanus (lockjaw) and strychnine poisoning, causing the body to assume a stiff position, especially the head, neck, ears, back, and tail. The mouth is closed as a result of contraction of masseter muscles, nostrils distended "trumpet like." Stiffness of the back without bending is called *orthotonus,* depression of spinal column and bending back of head toward withers, *opisthotonus,* spasms of the masseter muscles, *trismus,* spasms of the extensors of the limb, *sawhorse attitude,* muscles of the eye, *prolapsus of the membrana nictitans,* cramps of facial muscles, *risus sardonicus* (canine laugh). Tonic spasms in connection with clonic spasms are also observed in cerebro-spinal meningitis (*cramp of the neck*).

All spasms have their origin in the cortex of the cerebrum, the pyramidal tracts, or in the anterior cornua of the spinal cord. Spasms originating in the cerebrum are attended with mental disturbances (epilepsy), not so in case of *spinal spasms.*

Reflex spasms are due to irritation of peripheral sensory nerve endings and are of spinal origin; they are observed when animal parasites occur in the intestines, during the period of shedding teeth, and in painful gastric and intestinal affections.

b. **Involuntary movements** may be due to irritation of one of the cerebral hemispheres or to paralysis of the opposite one, also to affections of the midbrain or of the cerebellum. They always proceed from circumscribed lesions and are therefore known as "symptoms of local origin." Sometimes involuntary movements occur in the muscles of the body and extremities, or the usual voluntary movements assume an involuntary character. In such cases animals manifest a desire to "go ahead," trot with *head raised* or *lowered,* run against obstacles; if they get into a corner they are at a loss as to how to get out, frequently they fall down in such cases. Sometimes, but more rarely, they *walk backwards.* If the cerebral disturbances are unilateral the symptoms tend to be the same. The animals walk in a circle (*Reitbahnbewegungen, riding school movements:*) they lie down and roll, turning on their long axis, or they fix their hind feet as a pivot, and walk around with their forefeet—*move like the hands of a clock.* Involuntary movements are most frequently observed in chronic and acute hydrocephalus, abscesses, hemorrhages, tumors and parasites in the brain. Turn sickness, [gid], of sheep is thus characterized.

In so called riding school and clock hand movement the coenurus is usually located on the surface of that half of the cerebral hemisphere facing the center of the circle; sometimes on the optic thalamus of the opposite side.

If affected sheep move forward with the head down and trotting motion of the forelimbs (trotters) the seat of the parasite is at the anterior end of the hemisphere or on one of the corpora striata.

Staggering gait, reeling, dizziness (staggerers) indicate that the parasite is located in or on the cerebellum.

When the coenurus is located at the base of the cerebellum it causes *rolling* movements of the animal.

If the animals hold their heads up high or backwards and move forward rapidly, fall down (sailors), the coenurus is located in the posterior portion of the cerebrum.

c. **Disturbances of the muscular sense.** The muscular sense enables us to recognize the position of the limbs and the extent of passive and active movements. As long as equilibrium is not affected, an animal suffering from disease of the cerebrum can be made to assume unphysiologic positions without being conscious of it, in fact they do this themselves, they interrupt movements before they are completed or go to the opposite extreme and make more extensive movements than occur normally.

In acute cerebritis and staggers horses sometimes assume peculiar positions of the legs, cross them, set them close together or one before the other; one may be set unduly forward, the other unduly under the body. When such positions are produced passively the animals make no attempts to change them. In moving about they raise their legs unusually high, (groping, wading walk) or not high enough and thus *stumble* when they meet obstacles.

d. **Paralyses** consist in partial or complete loss of power to bring about muscular contractions. Complete inability to move is called *complete paralysis;* if there is simply diminished power to produce movements we call it *incomplete paralysis* (*paresis*). According to the origin of the paralysis we distinguish *cerebral, spinal,* and *peripheral* paralyses. Paralysis of one side of the body is called *hemi-*

plegia, of both sides (both hind legs) *paraplegia;* paralysis of a single organ or part is known as *monoplegia.* Hemiplegia has its origin in the brain, paraplegia in the spinal cord, monoplegia in the motor centers of the brain or, and as a rule, in peripheral nerves.

In cerebral paralyses the cranial nerves are frequently also affected and psychic disturbances are present; we observe cerebral paralysis in

1. Brain diseases: acute cerebritis, cerebro-spinal meningitis, abscesses, hemorrhages (apoplexies), tumors, parasites.
2. Infectious diseases: rabies, mal du coit (always), exceptionally in horse distemper, and in contagious pleuro-pneumonia of the horse.
3. In intoxication diseases: parturient fever, mycotic intoxications, brine poisoning.

Spinal paralyses are usually cases of paraplegia which affect all nerves beyond the point of injury or disease and are always attended with sensory paralysis. Psychic disturbances are wanting. They are caused by:

1. Spinal fractures;
2. Diseases of the cord: inflammation, hemorrhage, tumors, parasites;
3. Infectious diseases: dog distemper, rabies, rarely in contagious pleuro-pneumonia of the horse.

Spinal paralyses also affect the vegetative branch of the nervous system, since the lumbar cord is the center for the production of the contractions that produce defecation and urination. Hence paralysis of the rectum and bladder with the inevitable results (impaction of rectum and distention of bladder with urine) occurs. See pp. 137 *and* 148.

Peripheral paralyses are for the most part of surgical interest. In internal medicine paralysis of the facial nerve, because it interrupts normal feeding, and paralysis of the recurrent nerve, because it disturbs respiration, are of interest. These two morbid conditions have been considered more in detail elsewhere.

e. **Reflex excitability.** Reflex movement is a temporary muscular contraction brought about by stimulating a peripheral (sensory) nerve ending. In order that reflex movement may occur the sensory and motor nerve fibres and the reflex center must be intact. Reflex movement is limited to one muscle or muscle group (*simple reflex*) or it may affect the whole body and in that case may be *inco-ordinated (reflex spasm) or co-ordinated (motions of defense or flight)*. The following physiological reflexes are of clinical importance:

A. Reflexes of the Brain.

1. Closing of the eyelids. The sensory fibres (trigeminus) of the cornea, conjunctiva and of the skin in the neighborhood of the eye conduct impulses to the medulla oblongata and from that point the facial nerve produces contraction of the orbicularis of the eyelids.

2. Sensitiveness to light on part of the pupil. Stimulation of the optic nerve is transmitted reflexly, to the oculomotorius, which, through contraction of the sphincter pupillae, cause contraction of the pupil.

Increased reflex excitability occurs in tetanus and in strychnine poisoning. Contracted pupil is observed in morphine, eserine and pilocarpine poisoning.

Decreased reflex excitability in great mental depression, excessive pain and in dyspnea of high degree.

Dilated pupil (*mydriasis*) occurs in paralysis of the optic nerve (black cataract) and in paralysis of the oculo motor nerve (atropin poisoning).

B. Spinal Reflexes.

1. **Skin reflexes** consist of muscular contractions following irritation of sensory peripheral nerves, e. g. manipulation or percussion of the walls of the chest or the flank. Touching the anus causes contraction of the sphincter ani (anal reflex); touching the skin at the perineum results in drawing up of the tail and depression of the croup.

2. **Mucous membrane reflexes.** Pressure upon the larynx or the upper rings of the trachea produces a cough (laryngeal reflex).

3. **Tendon reflexes.** Striking the flexor tendons of the carpus, the inferior patellar ligaments or the achilles tendon causes the animal to raise its legs.

4. **Normal defecation and urination.**

Spinal reflexes are diminished or absent in disturbances of the reflex arc, hence in peripheral paralyses and diseases of the spinal cord. Increased reflexes are observed in hyperesthesia, strychnine poisoning and in diseases of the reflex inhibitory centers of the brain.

Diseases of the Nervous System.

Cerebral congestion. Hyperemia of short duration, fluctuating in character and entirely curable. Begins with stage of excitement; animals are restless, try to force themselves forward or sideways, rear, kick, shake their heads, walk backwards, tear the halter strap, etc. After a few hours the stage of depression sets in; animals are stupefied, sad look of the eye, head down, disregard familiar commands.

Acute cerebral anemia. Disturbance of consciousness, unsteady gait, staggering, leaning against objects for support, neighing, shaking of head, falling.

Acute inflammation of the brain, acute hydrocephalus. Differs from congestion in its more pronounced symptoms and its longer duration. In the second stage (that of depression), we observe abnormal attitudes and movements, staggering, sometimes falling down and inability to get up again, sometimes attacks of raving madness. Temperature frequently increased, but fever may be absent. Feeding always more or less interrupted, especially the **manner** of feeding

Blind staggers. Morosis equorum. Hydrocephalus chronicus. This is a chronic apyretic incurable affection of the cerebrum which manifests itself by mental disturbances, and by impaired locomotion and sensibility. Pulse strong and full, number of heart beats never increased, but frequently diminished—a very constant symptom. Appetite usually good but animal e a t s s l o w l y. Ability to work present to a limited degree. Examination for staggers.

Overheating (Hyperthermia) and **Sunstroke** (Insolatio). Exhaustion, dullness, unsteady gait; in the beginning, perspiration, abating and followed by increased bodily temperature. Death frequent, from cardiac paralysis.

Chorea. St. Vitus' Dance. Continuous, usually incoördinated, rarely apparently coördinated, involuntary, jerky movements of limbs or portions of the body.

Epilepsy. "Falling sickness" is a chronic disease of the brain characterized by paroxysms occuring at intervals and attended by sudden loss of consciousness and disturbed sensibility.

Dizziness, vertigo. This is a primary disease, occurring at intervals, characterized by interrupted equilibrium and due to circulatory disturbances in the brain.

Cerebral hemorrhage. Apoplexy. Sudden dizziness, involuntary movements, loss of consciousness, falling down, paralysis (hemiplegia and monoplegia).

Eclampsia is an acute epilepsy, ending in recovery or in death.

Turnsick is a disease of sheep caused by the presence of the larval form of Tenia coenurus in the brain. 1st stage, cerebral excitement; 2nd stage, latent stage; 3rd stage is that of turnsick, characterized by symptoms of local brain affections.

Paralysis of the facial nerve. In case of peripheral paralysis the cheeks, lips and nasal muscles are paralyzed, usually unilaterally; if paralysis is bilateral we have dyspnea and difficulty in feeding. In case of c e n t r a l paralysis the upper eyelids droop, eyes cannot be closed and the auricular muscles are affected.

Lumbar prurigo of sheep is a chronic, hereditary affection of the spinal cord characterized by hyperesthesia, weakness and paralysis of the hind parts and by progressive emaciation, invariably leads to death.

Infectious Diseases with Localization in the Central Nervous System.

Tetanus is an intoxication produced by the entrance of the products of the tetanus bacilli into the blood. Spasmodic condition of the entire skeletal muscles, animal is stiff, eyes retracted, membrana nictitans prolapsed, head and neck bent back, back depressed, tail erect. Sawhorse attitude of legs, hock turned out, producing bowleggedness. Spasm of masseter and pharyngeal muscles interfere with mastication and deglutition, spasm of the respiratory muscles affects respiration. Great excitability; thus aggravating the general muscular cramps. At first no fever, later on the fever is high. Pulse strong and full. Animals do not lie down, or when down they cannot get up. Mental condition is normal.

Rabies is a strictly infectious disease characterized by disturbance of the central nervous system. 1. Initial stage. Dogs are restless, moody, easily frightened, want to be out of doors, depraved appetite. 2. Raving stage. Aimless running about, tendency to bite, sometimes break their own teeth in the act, voice changed to a barking howl. 3. Paralytic stage. Emaciation, lower jaw paralyzed, tongue extended, hind quarters paralyzed. Horses show restlessness as in colic, neigh in a peculiar shrill or yelling manner, try to gnaw or bite the point of infection, bite the manger and not infrequently fracture the lower jaw in the act. Paralysis and death follow within three days. Cattle bellow and run against objects with their horns, frequently fracturing them. Sheep and pigs also manifest a desire to bite.

Infectious cerebro-spinal meningitis. Disease is frequently introduced with chills. Slight fever. Sensibility reduced, animals are drowsy, stumble and fall on slight provocation. Turning of eyes, jerking of muscles, later on paralysis. Tonic spasms of the cervical muscles; head drawn to one side.

Tuberculosis of the Brain. Irregular movements of the head or unusual position. Jerky movements and spasms. Frequent and continuous lateral decubitus. Inability to rise. Symptoms sometimes acute.

Intoxication Diseases.

Parturient paresis, milk fever, is an acute auto-intoxication closely following the act of parturition, and characterized by cerebral paralysis. Begins with slight, temporary, cerebral excitement;

after a few hours symptoms of depression and paralysis set in. Animals lie immovably in a characteristic attitude, see p. 34. Eyes closed, paralysis of muscles of head, tongue extended, rattling breathing, distention of abdomen, constipation, paresis of paunch. Lowering of external and internal bodily temperature.

C. Specific Examinations.

We resort to the specific examinations only when definite results cannot be obtained with the foregoing methods, especially in cases of differential diagnosis between similar diseases. In all cases the specific examinations are directed toward determining definite diseases; and the characteristics of these are specially considered.

12. Body Movements.

Many diseases are not observed until the animal is in harness or under the saddle, others become more conspicuous in their symptoms under these conditions. The rule is to examine animals while engaged in their accustomed occupation (blind staggers, balkiness). Draft horses should be examined when hitched to the wagon, riding horses under their rider. Unaccustomed work fatigues animals unduly and excites them. Sometimes fatigue and excitement make certain symptoms more conspicuous (roaring) ; in such cases we make an exception of the rule just given. In all cases we must observe that the animal is properly harnessed.

I. Examination for Immobility.
(Examination of So-called Dummies).

Blind Staggers.

Blind staggers may be defined as an incurable disease of the brain accompanied by cerebral depression. It may develop gradually or follow an attack of acute hydrocephalus. Accordingly, blind staggers is characterized by disturbances of consciousness. These symptoms may be observed while the animal is at rest, but frequently they are not sufficiently pronounced so that a diagnosis can be based upon them. Subjecting a suspicious animal to exercise is a valuable aid in making a diagnosis, it furnishes a better opportunity for testing the psychic functions and the resulting increased blood pressure intensifies the existing symptoms.

It is of diagnostic importance that horses affected with immobility can be used for work, though in a limited degree, and that horses suffering with acute cerebral affections refuse to work or, if worked, *symptoms of cerebral excitement follow*. Again, horses with blind staggers always have a low pulse, eat *slowly* but nevertheless *eat a full feed*. On the other hand, horses with acute cerebral affections have poor appetite and a high, or changeable, pulse.

In examining for blind staggers the horses must be tested while performing accustomed duties, and care must be observed not to excite them; in no case must they be subjected to unaccustomed work. It is advisable to drive or ride the animal oneself; notice the facility with which the animal is guided, effect of whip and spurs, tendency to go over to one side, ease with which animal moves forward or backward. As soon as the animal *begins to sweat* it is taken to a quiet place and rested, here we repeat a careful examination of the *cerebral functions*, (the animal's psychical condition); observe the expression of the eye, effect of surroundings, general attitude of the body, movements of the head, use of eyes and ears. To determine the degree of sensibility we resort to mechanical irritation: gently inserting a finger into the animal's ear, flipping the finger against the nose, stepping on the coronet, kicking against the cannon bone. Finally the animal's motility is tested to determine whether it voluntarily assumes unnatural positions (setting a foot abnormally forward or back) whether it advances or *backs* readily, follows its leader or not, halts without a command when the attendant leading it stops, etc. An important test is to

Fig. 52.

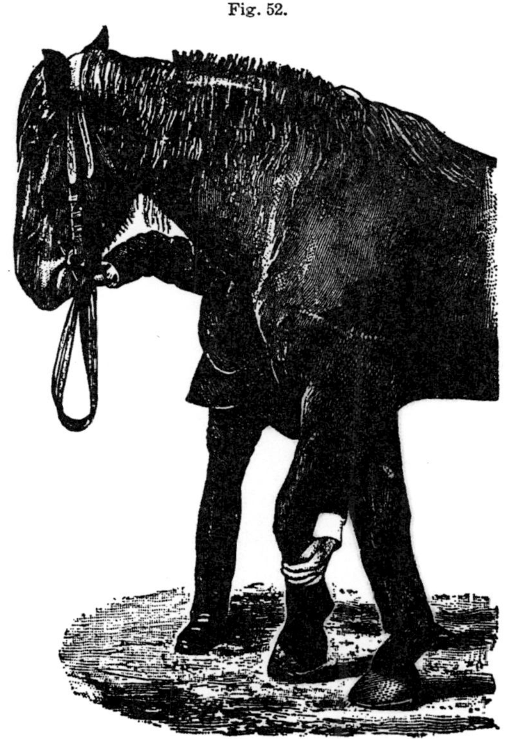

Examination of a horse for Blind Staggers.

attempt to cross the forelegs; horses with blind staggers can usually be made to assume this position and throw their weight on their feet when thus crossed. To make this test the operator stands on one side of the animal, his legs spread so that one is in front, and the other behind the front leg of the horse, then grasps the foot of the opposite side (at the metacarpus and from behind), forces the horse back a little to relieve the foot in question, pulls it over and crosses it in front of its opposite.

Quiet and gentle animals will sometimes remain standing in this position and even permit other insults, but from their general attitude it is plain that the reason for all this is not an abnormal mental state but rather extreme good naturedness. Animals greatly fatigued may show symptoms of a depressed sensorium, but they are always of short duration.

A single symptom can never determine a diagnosis, we must consider the animal's condition as a whole.

II. Examination for Heaves.

Heaves may be defined as a chronic, incurable disease of the lungs or of the heart, characterized by difficult and laborious respiration.

This definition is forensic in its sense, and includes a number of chronic incurable diseases of the lungs and of the heart that are attended with difficult respiration. As a rule chronic bronchitis, alveolar emphysema of the lungs, chronic interstitial pneumonia or heart disease constitute the anatomical lesion at the bottom of *heaves*. Although it is frequently possible to determine the exact nature of the anatomical lesion, it is customary, in Germany at least, to apply the term "heaves" to all of these conditions, because "heaves" is considered as one of those diseases the presence of which is a legal ground for the setting aside of a contract of sale and is referred to under this name in all laws concerning it.

The term "difficult and laborious respiration" is comparative in its sense, and in applying it we must always consider the nature of the exercise leading to it as well as the constitution and anatomical make-up of the animal. On the other hand, whether the pathological condition in any way affects the use of the animal for some particular purpose or not, does not come under consideration. To make a positive diagnosis of "heaves" it is necessary only to recognize the existence of a difficulty of respiration which is due to a chronic and incurable disease of the lungs or of the heart.

For this purpose a careful examination of the circulatory apparatus and of the respiratory apparatus is indispensable. It is also necessary to determine *positive* symptoms of the disorder under consideration in order to be fortified against the possible assertion that the disease is due to other causes than chronic and incurable affections of the lungs or of the heart. Furthermore, we must exclude, by careful examination of all functional apparatus, any acute affections that may produce increased respiration. External painful conditions must also be taken into consideration.

If it is impossible to differentiate between the effects of disturbances of this nature and existing symptoms of heaves, it would be well, in all cases where legal complications are possible, to inform both buyer and seller of the existing conditions and of the necessity of withholding the expression of a final opinion until the animal has recovered from the existing acute disease. If, at such a time, the previously observed symptoms of "heaves" are still present, the existence of the disease at the time of purchase must be conceded.

The examination of a suspected "heavey" horse is conducted not only while the animal is at rest, but also during and after exercise. Animals are worked in an accustomed manner and made to exert themselves to a moderate degree, at the same time we note the character and frequency of respiration. The horse should be driven or ridden in a quiet trot; a draft horse made to pull a moderately heavy load. Count the respirations every 5 minutes and let the animal work until it sweats, but not longer than 15 minutes. Then put the animal in a stable, count the respirations every 5 minutes and note when they return to the normal (the number counted before exercising).

In healthy horses the number of respirations runs as high as 50 or 70 per minute, sometimes even higher. Respiration occurs without exertion, the animals may now and then give a voluntary snort and take a few deep inspirations. In the course of at most 15 to 18 minutes after cessation of the exercise, the number of respirations should be reduced to that observed at rest.

"Heavey" horses, on the other hand, show increased or difficult breathing, dyspnea (see p. 99). Inspiration and expiration may be so difficult that the number is not increased, but the character of the respiratory movements enables us to recognize the dyspnea. But as a rule the number of respirations, when animals are exercised as above described, runs up to 80 to 120 per minute and goes back to the normal very gradually. Not infrequently this requires 30 to 60 minutes. In chronic bronchitis a white foamy nasal discharge is observed.

III. Examination for Roaring.

The term "roaring" is applied to a form of breathing attended with the production of an audible sound and due to a chronic, incurable disease of the larynx or trachea.

As a rule, roaring is caused by a paralysis of the left recurrent nerve and the resulting inactivity and degeneration of the muscles which it supplies (*Hemiplegia laryngis sinistra*).

In rare cases a paralysis of the right recurrent nerve or a bilateral paralysis may exist; sometimes thickening of the mucous membrane or the presence of tumors may be the cause. An exact diagnosis of the cause of such a stenosis can be definitely determined only with the aid of the laryngoscope; but in 99 per cent. of all cases a left handed paralysis is the cause.

Except in rare cases, laryngeal roaring is noticed only in forcible or increased respiration, and is then characterized by a harsh, sharp inspiratory noise or tone (wheezing, whistling, blowing, humming, roaring, snoring.) The respiratory noise is caused by the fact that deep and rapid inspiration causes the air current to force the paralyzed arytenoid cartilage and vocal cord into the lumen of the larynx and thus obstructs its free passage. Decreasing the volume of the ingoing current of air by compressing the nostrils causes the noise to cease. Pressure on the paralyzed arytenoid cartilage increases the noise. Pressure on the right (unaffected) cartilage increases dyspnoea to such an extent that inspiration is almost impossible, it ceases entirely or continues with a sharp wheezing sound, because the lumen of the larynx is now obstructed by both arytenoid cartilages.

In examining for roaring the horse must be placed under conditions that force it to make rapid and energetic respiratory movements, it must be "worked hard," pull heavy loads over soft ground, or gallop. Exercising or riding are especially adapted for this purpose because we can control the position of the head, and thus influence respiration. Whether or not the animal is accustomed to this sort of exercise has no effect on the general result.

If the head and neck of the animal are well checked up and back, the points of insertion of the dorsal muscles are approximated and the action of the latter on the spinal column is reduced: now, in order to fix the spinal column the longissimus dorsi, the inspiratory and the abdominal muscles must be contracted with unusual force; this can be done only at the moment of inspiration. In expiration these muscles are relaxed and the animal loses, more or less, the control over its spinal column. It therefore makes an effort to reduce the expiratory period by rapidly and energetically following with the inspiratory movement. If only one arytenoid cartilage projects over the lumen of the larynx the inspiratory current forces it in, produces a stenosis and causes the respiratory sound. By turning the head toward the right the in-streaming current of air is directed on the left arytenoid cartilage, and if the paralysis is only an incomplete one the characteristic sound is produced just the same.

This kind of treatment can never produce roaring in a healthy horse.

In order to make a positive diagnosis of "roaring" it is necessary to eliminate the possible presence of acute morbid conditions of the upper air passages as well as stenoses of the nasal cavities since these conditions will also produce audible breathing. Contractions or other deformities of the nasal cavities can frequently be recognized upon superficial examination, or by the wheezing noise they produce. If the trouble is unilateral, the peculiar noise will cease upon closing the affected side, or become more pronounced upon obstruction of the healthy nostril.

If existing lameness or the presence of acute affections of the respiratory apparatus or other organs make this method of examination impossible, the laryngoscope may do valuable service.

IV. Examination for Epilepsy and Vertigo.

Epilepsy is a chronic cerebral disease that is characterized by paroxysms occurring at intervals and attended with interruption or loss of consciousness and sensibility. Vertigo (dizziness) is a similar affection; it is an independent disease occurring in the form of periodical attacks, disturbed equilibrium and consciousness. The difference between epilepsy and vertigo is that spasms are absent in the latter.

The diagnosis of these two diseases is not difficult if one has an opportunity to observe an *attack*. In the intervals horses act perfectly normal. Sometimes certain known conditions bring about an attack; when making an examination of suspected animals we can often make use of this knowledge to bring on an attack. Horses may be hitched up and driven as on former occasions when an attack was observed, etc. The fit of the harness should be carefully inspected. Sometimes frightening or exciting the animal, or driving with the face turned toward the setting sun, or along streets sprinkled with alternating shade of trees and the glaring light of the sun, will produce an attack. If we cannot personally observe an attack we must base our diagnosis upon unobjectionable statements of witnesses.

Epilepsy. Characteristic epileptic spasms occur either only at the head and neck (partial epilepsy) or the whole body is affected (general epilepsy). Animals stop suddenly, distort their eyes, blink, spasmodically contract the muscles of the lips and face, raise their heads high and jerk them to one side, sometimes they step to and fro, or backward and forward, restlessly. In general epilepsy the spasms rapidly extend over the whole body; masticatory movements are spasmodic, the saliva is churned into foam, the animals grate their teeth, spasmodically distort their neck sideways, the muscles generally undergo spasmodic contractions, the animals stagger and fall and then the spasms may continue for some minutes. An attack may last from ¼ to 15 minutes, the horses then get up and become quieted. The intervals between attacks are very irregular.

The above described idiopathic epilepsy must be distinguished from acute cerebral affections and from epileptiform spasms due to peripheral irritations (reflex epilepsy).

Vertigo. Attacks usually occur while animals are at work; they suddenly walk slower, nod and shake their heads, snort, raise their heads up and sideways, stagger, spread their legs and not infrequently fall down. Here they lie quietly, sometimes kick a little and then get up again. During the attack there is a loss of consciousness and sensibility, sometimes increased respiration and profuse sweating.

Attacks of dizziness due to congestion of the brain (compression of the jugulars) and to cerebral anemia (stenosis of aortic valves) do not belong under the head of idiopathic vertigo.

V. Examination for Balkiness.

Balkiness is refractoriness manifested in common and accustomed work. Hence a horse must be tested while at *accustomed* work, and we must proceed with utmost caution and quiet and avoid everything that might excite the animal. The examining veterinarian must be present during all manipulations and see to it that rough or improper treatment is avoided.

We first examine those parts of the body that bear the weight and pressure of the harness and see that no morbid or painful conditions exist; the animal is then properly harnessed. In case the harness does not fit, it should be made so by shortening or lengthening parts that may require it, or by using a new set of harness. Then the animal is tested in the capacity for which it is intended, single or double, as coach or draft horse, or under the rider, as the case may be. Active or passive refractoriness to reasonable demands is regarded as *balkiness*.

Young animals, such as are not yet sufficiently accustomed to work, also evince a certain degree of refractoriness, but, as a rule, if properly handled they will soon yield and obey willingly, especially if they are hitched with older and quiet horses.

13. Diagnostic Inoculation.

Diagnostic inoculations consist in the introduction of certain substances into the bodies of animals for the purpose of determining either the character of the substance or the condition of the animal's health. We base our judgment on the character of the result. For the clinician diagnostic inoculations serve merely to recognize a few infectious diseases; certain of these diseases have so rapid a course that the clinical symptoms cannot be relied upon to determine either their kind or character with any degree of certainty. Others which terminate much less rapidly do not show sufficient symptoms for a definite diagnosis. In these cases nothing save a correctly performed inoculation will serve to recognize the disease or to obtain an early diagnosis.

Diagnostic inoculations are always made with respect to certain well known infectious diseases which our examination leads us to suspect. In performing the inoculation, therefore, we must consider the peculiarities of these diseases, we choose certain tissues, fluids or other substances for our inoculating material, we follow a certain method of inoculation and make use of particular animals.

For inoculation we use

1. Material of known composition (tuberculin, mallein) in order to determine the condition of the animals from the resulting reaction.
2. Tissue and other material from diseased an-

imals on test or experimental animals in order to determine the pathogenic character of the inoculated material.

Diagnostic inoculations are of particular value in the infectious diseases which follow.

I. Tuberculosis.

Tuberculosis can be recognized in only a small per cent. of affected animals by the use of ordinary clinical methods.

On the one hand only a few symptoms can be determined, on the other hand these symptoms are not characteristic because they also occur in other diseases. The discovery of the tubercle bacillus as the cause of tuberculosis is hardly of any value in the clinical diagnosis of the disease in animals. Morbid products from an affected organ (lung of cow) for microscopical examination, are difficult to obtain; the quantity is small and besides is swallowed by the animal as soon as it reaches the pharynx. But, an opportunity to examine pathological nasal secretions, ejections, vaginal discharges or pathologically altered milk must never be neglected. (See p. 94.)

Under these circumstances the experimental determination of this disease is of great importance. For this purpose we resort to the tuberculin test and to the inoculation of small experimental animals.

The tuberculin test. Tuberculin is the toxin of the tubercle bacilli, obtained from artificial cultures of the same. The tubercle bacilli are cultivated for six weeks in 5% glycerine beef bouillon at 38° C. [100.4° F.] The culture is then sterilized at 110°C. [230° F.] and filtered through unglazed porcelain tubes. The filtrate is evaporated to one-tenth its volume and thus constitutes tuberculin. After these manipulations the tuberculin is absolutely free from germs and therefore it could never produce tuberculosis. Furthermore, it has no permanent injurious influence on either sick or healthy animals.

Dose.* The tuberculin prepared as above described is diluted with 9 volumes of water to which ½% of carbolic acid has been added. Cattle and horses receive 5 cc of this solution, yearlings 2.5 cc, calves 1 cc and dogs 0.5—1cc.

Technique. The tuberculin is injected subcutaneously at the neck or in front of the shoulder. Before and after using, the hypodermic syringe should be disinfected with a 2% solution of carbolic acid. Before inserting the hypodermic needle smooth down the hair at the point of injection. Disinfection of the injected area is not necessary if care is exercised otherwise. The best time for injection is in the evening between 9 and 10 o'clock. The bodily temperature of the animal to be injected should have been ascertained at noon of the day of injection and also just before injection. Eight or nine hours after injection of the tuberculin, hence at 6 A. M., next day, the temperature of each animal should again be taken, and thereafter every two hours until the 18th hour after injection. Perhaps it is unnecessary to state that the temperatures should be recorded.

Interpretation of Results. In tuberculous animals the injection of tuberculin produces fever (reaction), healthy animals are not affected.

a. Cattle with pre-injection temperatures *not* exceeding 39.5° C. [103.1° F.] and post-injection temperatures exceeding 39.5° C. [103.1° F.], providing the difference between the highest pre-injection temperature and the highest post-injection temperature is at least 1° C. [1.8° F.] are regarded as tuberculous.

b. In calves under 6 months of age a rise of temperature exceeding 40° C. (104° F.) after injection of the tuberculin,

[*This applies, of course, to the German tuberculin. In America the article is manufactured by a number of reliable firms. It should always be used as fresh as possible and the dose regulated according to the strength of the material. This is always indicated in the "directions for use."]

provided the difference between the highest pre- and post-injunction temperatures is at least 1° C. (1.8° F.) indicates the existence of tuberculosis.

The International Veterinary Congress of Budapest has accepted the following interpretation of the results of a tuberculin test:

1. A *post-injection* temperature exceeding 40° C. [104° F.], provided the temperature at the time of injection did not exceed 39.5° C. (103.1° F.), is to be regarded as a positive reaction.

In *post-injection* temperatures of cattle between 39.5° C. [103.1° F.] and 40° C. [104.0° F.] the results are to be regarded as doubtful and to be considered upon their own merits.

If the *pre-injection* temperatures of cattle exceed 39.5° C. [103.1° F.], or if those of calves less than six months of age exceed 40° C. [104.0° F.], the tuberculin test should be made at a later date.

Reliability. The tuberculin test cannot be regarded as absolutely infallible. About 95% of the tuberculous animals give a positive reaction. Animals in advanced stage of the disease frequently do not react. As a rule, however, a physical examination of such animals reveals symptoms which, when considered alone, would at least awaken suspicion as to the existence of the disease. Only a small per cent. of the reacting animals is found to be free from tuberculosis. Nevertheless, tuberculin is the best diagnosticum in our possession.

The Conjunctival or Ophthalmic Tuberculin Test. With a camel's hair brush or by means of a pipette introduce one-half cubic centimeter of common tuberculin, tuberculin A, or Bovo-Tuberculol D, solutio I, into the conjunctival sac. To facilitate the operation, secure the head of the animal, depress the lower eyelid and drop the tuberculin into the pocket thus formed.

Tuberculosis is indicated if a pronounced mucopurulent conjunctivitis develops in a few hours.

The technic is simple and may be carried out without securing the animals.

Results thus far have not been uniformly the same, but are nearly as reliable as those obtained from the Subcutaneous Method. The positive reactions are more trustworthy than the negative.

The Intracutaneous Method.

On a smooth healthy portion of the side of the neck, locate two points separated by a distance of five centimeters. These points should be marked for identification by clipping the hair. Place the thumb and index finger of the left hand on these points, draw the skin into a fold and ascertain the thickness of the fold by means of a suitable instrument. Clean the skin between the two points with alcohol, raise the same into a longitudinal fold and then inject into the cutis O. 1 cm. of a mixture of equal parts of tuberculin and normal physiological salt solution. Use a graduated syringe and a fine needle.

If the swelling of the skin increases 0.3 cm. or more in the course of twenty-four hours, the animal is to be regarded as tuberculous. Slight swellings or premature swellings are of doubtful significance.

The cutaneous tuberculin test is not as reliable as either of the foregoing.

These so-called local tests are recommended when the temperature of the animal is abnormally high or when variations occur or are suspected. Sometimes the application of several methods is of value. The local tests may be applied simultaneously and then followed by the subcutaneous.

Inoculation of Experimental Animals. The milk of tuberculous animals contains tubercle bacilli in all cases where the udder is affected with tubercular processes; frequently also in the apparent absence of such processes. The udder should be thoroughly milked, massaged and then again milked. The last drawing of milk is centrifuged, the cream and sediment mixed and used for intraperitoneal injection. If tubercle bacilli are present, tubercular nodules will develop on the peritoneum (omentum), spleen and liver in the course of two weeks. Unless the innoculated animals die before, they should be killed at the end of six weeks and examined for lesions of tuberculosis.

According to Ostertag, the innoculations are best made at the posterior inner surface of the thigh. This produces results much sooner than the intraperitoneal method. Pseudo tubercular processes are also avoided by this means. Experimental animals may be killed for bacteriological examination as soon as the lymph glands become conspicuous as painless circumscribed tumors. This may occur in the course of ten days, otherwise the animals should be killed for examination by the end of the sixth week.

II. Glanders.

In view of the great infectiousness and incurability of glanders, the object of the veterinarian is to determine the presence or absence of this disease at the earliest possible date. However, horses affected with glanders show no symptoms or at least no characteristic symptoms in the early stages of the disease; for this reason horses that have been exposed to an infection with glanders are subjected to a mallein test, with the object of thus enabling us to recognize the disease. If the animals show symptoms of the disease we endeavor to obtain some of the pathological products or secretions and with them inoculate experimental animals which are known from experience to be susceptible to the disease and develop it in a characteristic form.

Mallein inoculation. Mallein is the toxin of the bacilli of glanders and is obtained from their cultures in a manner analogous to that employed for obtaining tuberculin. The crude preparation is a fluid, obtainable from the manufacturer and injected in doses designated. It may also be obtained in the dry or powdered form and is thus injected in doses of 0.02—0.1 G. according to the weight of the animal. It is best to have the solution of the dry tuberculin prepared by the manufacturer.

T e c h n i q u e. This is the same as for tuberculin inoculation. Taking temperature of animal to be tested, two or three times at definite intervals before inoculation; inoculation between 10-12 P. M., and taking temperatures again on next day beginning at 5 A. M., and repeating every two hours until 6 P. M.

Interpretation of Results. The International Veterinary Congress has accepted the following principles for guidance in interpreting the results of a mallein test:

1. A positive reaction to mallein confirms the diagnosis of glanders only when it possesses a typical character.

2. A typical reaction consists of an elevation of temperature of at least two degrees centigrade [3.8° F.] and must exceed 40° C. [104° F.] The temperature curve usually remains at an elevation for some time or it may make a slight drop and rise again on the same day. On the second, and sometimes on the third day, there will be more or less elevation of temperature. A local as well as a general or constitutional reaction is also observed.

3. Elevations of temperature less than 40° C. [104° F.], as well as greater elevations of an atypical character require re-testing of the animal.

4. Gradually attained high temperatures of considerable duration, even if not typical, indicate the existence of glanders.

5. A local typical infiltration of the tissues at the point of inoculation is a positive indication of the existence of glanders, even in cases where no thermal or general organic reaction occurs.

6. All malleinized animals, whether they react or not, must be subjected to the mallein test twice, at intervals of ten to twenty days.

The results of the mallein test cannot be compared with those of the tuberculin test; they are less reliable. There is no doubt that the varying results obtained from the use of mallein are due to differences in the character of the mallein used.

Serum Diagnosis by Means of Agglutination.

The term Agglutinate is used to designate the characteristic of Blood Serum, which enables it to precipitate living as well as dead bacteria in the form of clumps. The active elements in this process are called Agglutinines. The normal blood serum of the horse agglutinates glanders bacilli in a limited degree. However, if a horse is affected with glanders, the agglutinines appear in larger masses.

In order to make an Agglutination Test for glanders, the serum of the blood of the suspected horse is prepared in various dilutions by means of the addition of a physiological salt solution. In order to determine the agglutinating power, equal quantities of emulsions of glanders bacilli which have been destroyed by heating at 60°C. (test fluid) are added to the serum solutions.

Horses, the blood serum of which will agglutinate glanders bacilli in dilutions of 1:1000 or in greater dilutions, must be regarded as affected with glanders. Agglutinating powers ranging from 1:500 to 1000 are doubtful. Agglutinating powers in dilutions of 1:400 to 500 indicate the absence of glanders. Exceptions occur in all of these cases. In case of doubtful results, the test must be repeated after the lapse of a certain period of time.

The real weakness of the agglutination test consists on the one hand in the fact that horses that have chronic glanders frequently have a very low agglutinating power and, on the other hand, healthy horses sometimes possess an agglutinating power as high as that usually found in glandered horses.

Since it is the *degree* of agglutination and not agglutination itself that determines whether or not infection is present, the misinterpretations of results are unavoidable. Of course we can use for comparison such results only as have been produced by the same test fluid.

Inoculation of experimental animals. A male Guinea pig is inoculated subcutaneously at the abdomen with nasal secretion, pus, etc., from a suspicious subject. If the inoculated material contains the bacilli of glanders a local abscess will develop at the point of inoculation and a firm hot swelling appear in the region of the thigh. After 2-4 weeks the Guinea pig is killed with chloroform. The presence of the characteristic nodules, etc., of glanders, in the region of the point of inoculation and in the testicles confirms the diagnosis.

The method of Strauss, consisting of the intra-peritoneal inoculation of male Guinea pigs, is of more recent introduction. With a cotton swab dip up some of the suspicious material from an ulcer or from nasal secretion, rinse in a few cubic centimeters of sterilized water, and inject one or two cubic centimeters of this fluid into the abdominal cavity of each of several Guinea pigs. If the inoculated material contained the bacilli of glanders, reddening and swelling of the scrotum and adhesion of the testicles will occur in the course of two or three days. More or less isolated pus centers develop on the tunica vaginalis and cause an adhesion of the peritoneal folds. Sometimes a single center at the point of inoculation, constitutes the only lesion. The danger of a general septic infection, from the impure material, may be obviated by keeping the infected swabs in a refrigerator for a few days. Potato cultures should always be made from the lesions of the scrotum. The true glanders bacillus produces yellow colonies resembling honey in color, while the pseudobacillus of glanders (Kutscher) produces white colonies.

Cats, also, are suitable animals for inoculation. They are inoculated at the back of the neck.

Serum Diagnosis by Means of Complement Fixation. In glandered horses the toxin (antigen) of the glanders bacilli causes the formation of antibodies. These antibodies can develop only in the body of an animal affected with glanders. Fresh Guinea pig serum contains free complements which, with the aid of the glanders antibodies, have the power to fix the antigen. This fixing power is increased by heating the mixture at 37°C. in a thermostat. The diagnosis of glanders by this method consists in the determination of the amount of antibodies of glanders bacilli in the blood of a suspected horse.

The blood serum of a rabbit, when the latter has been treated with red blood corpuscles of the sheep, contains an antibody (hemolytic amboceptor) which will dissolve sheep blood corpuscles if free complement is added.

If, therefore, we add free complement (fresh Guinea pig serum) to the blood serum of a glandered horse and then add rabbit serum containing hemolytic amboceptor, this mixture, if added to the red blood corpuscles of the sheep, will leave the latter intact, because the complement that was added was already fixed to the antigen by means of the glanders antibodies. Now, the blood serum of healthy horses does not contain these antibodies and consequently the complement added to it does not become fixed, but remains active. This free complement, with the hemolytic antibody, dissolves the corpuscles of the blood in healthy horses.

The technique of serum diagnosis by means of complement fixation is as follows: To a measured quantity of blood serum from a suspected glandered horse add glanders antigen and fresh Guinea pig serum (this contains free complement), then heat at 37°C. in a thermostat for a few hours. Then add serum from a treated rabbit (as explained above) and also some thoroughly washed red blood corpuscles from a sheep. If the red corpuscles thus added are not dissolved the horse is affected with glanders. If they are dissolved the horse in question is free from the disease.

This method of diagnosis can be accurately conducted in specially equipped laboratories only, and is therefore not adapted for use by the regular practitioner. It is practicable, however, for the latter to collect the blood of the suspected horse and transmit it for examination.

III. Anthrax, Blackleg, Malignant Oedema and Wild-und Rinder-seuche.

On account of their rapid course, the clinical diagnosis of these diseases is often impossible; besides, the symptoms of the different diseases are often much alike and hence a differentiation impossible. Although a microscopical examination of the blood (or exudate) of animals that died of one of these diseases suffices to recognize their character by finding the characteristic organisms, still there are cases where an inoculation alone can decide the question. We use rabbits for this purpose and inoculate them cutaneously (!) in the ear, with blood or exudate from the animal or carcass in question. If the rabbit dies the disease is either anthrax or Wildseuche because blackleg and malignant oedema are not transmissible by means of cutaneous inoculation. The differentiation between anthrax and Wildseuche is made by a bacterioscopic examination of the dead rabbit. It is also worthy of note that in Wildseuche there is always a severe tracheitis.

In case the rabbit does not die, it is again inoculated; this time subcutaneously; if death follows, it was a case of malignant oedema because rabbits are immune against blackleg. The presence of blackleg can be demonstrated by inoculating a Guinea pig with the suspected material; death following in a few days after inoculation.

We can expedite matters by simultaneously inoculating one rabbit cutaneously and another rabbit and a Guinea pig subcutaneously. If all three animals die we had anthrax (or Wildseuche) if only the two subcutaneously inoculated animals die it was a case of malignant oedema, and in case it was blackleg only one animal, the Guinea pig, is sacrificed.

*If we desire additional proof by having the blood of a suspected anthrax carcass examined by a second person we may boil a potato, upon cooling cut it in halves with a steri-

* [This method is commonly resorted to in Germany.]

lized (flamed) knife, apply some of the suspected material to the surface of one half, replace the other half, pack carefully and send it to the official bacteriologist. Blood sent in a flask, is usually not adapted for microscopical examination.

IV. Rabies.

Suspected dogs are usually killed before they can be subjected to examination by an expert. A post mortem examination will then hardly enable us to make a definite positive diagnosis; we must resort to inoculation of a test animal. The diagnostic inoculation of a rabbit with the brain matter of a suspected dog is the only absolutely safe method of definitely determining the presence of rabies.

Technique. The brain and cervical cord of the suspected dog are carefully removed. The medulla oblongata is severed from the brain by an incision, at the pons Varolii, made with a "flamed" knife. A piece of the medulla (size of a pea) is removed with sterilized scissors from the cut surface, placed into a sterilized porcelain vessel and thoroughly triturated with a small quantity of distilled water. This emulsion is used for inoculation.

1. **The Intra-ocular method according to Johne.** Two rabbits are inoculated, each receiving a few drops of the emulsion into the anterior chamber of the eye; injected with a sterilized hypodermic syringe. If the hypodermic needle is fine and sharp and the rabbit's eye has been previously disinfected and anesthetized the operation can be performed with little difficulty. We insert the needle at the border of the cornea, directing it toward the median line. If the operation was carefully conducted a slight turbidity of the cornea, which soon disappears, is the only symptom that follows.

If rabies is present the first symptoms appear in from 2 weeks to 23 days; the animals are shy, crawl away, and show loss of appetite. After 12 hours paralysis and difficult deglutition is observed, the animals emaciate rapidly, grit their teeth and emit a cry when touched on the head. The disease, thus produced, terminates fatally within 48 hours.

2. Subdural Inoculation. Carefully trephine the frontal bone of a rabbit, observing the necessary antiseptic and anatomical precautions. By means of a sterilized glass syringe having its nozzle bent at right angles, inject a few drops of the emulsion under the duramater, stitch the wound and protect with collodion, or absorbent cotton.

If the inoculation material is fresh and virulent, death will follow in two or three weeks. Sometimes the animals die as early as the 11th day, or may live until the 30th day. [In some cases six weeks will elapse before the first symptoms of the disease can be observed.]

3. Intra-muscular Inoculation. If the suspected nerve tissue has begun to decompose, or if suspicion exists that it may not be fresh, it should be immersed in a one-half per cent. solution of carbolic acid and placed in the refrigerator for 24 hours. It is then removed and carefully triturated with beef broth until a fine emulsion results. Rabbits receive from three to five cubic centimeters of this emulsion injected into the dorsal muscles in the region of the loins. As a rule septic infection can be avoided in this way while the virulence of the material is otherwise unaffected. Death follows after two or three weeks or somewhat later.

The symptoms following subdural and intra-muscular inoculation are much the same. After ten or twelve days emaciation sets in, followed by paralysis of the hind parts, and death two or three days later.

4. Subconjunctival Inoculation. This is recommended by Szpilman as easy of execution and certain in its results.

In the "Tollwuthabteilung of the Institut fuer Infectionskrankheiten," in Berlin, the subdural and the intra-muscular inoculations are used exclusively, sometimes both methods are used at the same time. (Beck).

Differential diagnosis. Beck calls attention to the fact that material obtained from dogs affected with the nervous form of distemper will produce paralysis of the hind parts of rabbits that have been inoculated. In these cases the paralysis is not confined to the posterior extremities, but extends to the bladder and rectum. Rabbits thus affected become soiled with feces and urine. This affection cannot be transmitted to a second generation of rabbits.

14. The Lymphatic Glands.

The intermaxillary lymphatic glands of horses are always subjected to an examination in diseases of the respiratory apparatus. Otherwise they are subjected to *special examinations* only when infectious diseases, *glanders and tuberculosis*, constitutional blood diseases (*leucemia*) or the presence of malignant tumors (*carcinoma and sarcoma*) are suspected. Examination consists in palpation (conducted according to the rules given on p. 21). The correct interpretation of these changes was discussed under "intermaxillary lymphatic glands."

When an examination is called for, the following *lymphatic glands* must be considered:

1. *Intermaxillary lymphatic glands, lympho-glandula submaxillaris.* In the ox these are of the size of half a walnut and are situated on the median side of the submaxilla, near its border and in the region of the point of insertion of the musc. sterno-maxillaris.

2. *Lymphatic glands of the parotid region, lymphoglandula parotideae.* These are between and below the lobules of the parotid gland. In the ox they have the shape of a flattened tongue and a length approaching 6cm.; this gland projects from beneath the border of the parotid gland, below the maxillary articulation.

3. *The superior cervical glands lymphoglandula cervicales superiores, and retropharyngeales* are situated, as the name implies, on the posterior wall of the pharynx. In the ox they consist of a closely united packet, about 5cm. long, under the lateral processes of the atlas, where they can be felt by placing the thumb on the lateral

process of the atlas (both sides simultaneously) and thus pressing the finger tips behind the pharynx and then against the inferior face of the lateral processes of the atlas.

4. In the ox a few large lymph follicles in the depression in front of the shoulder (prescapular glands) and on the chest in front of the elbow articulation (prepectoral glands).

Fig. 53.

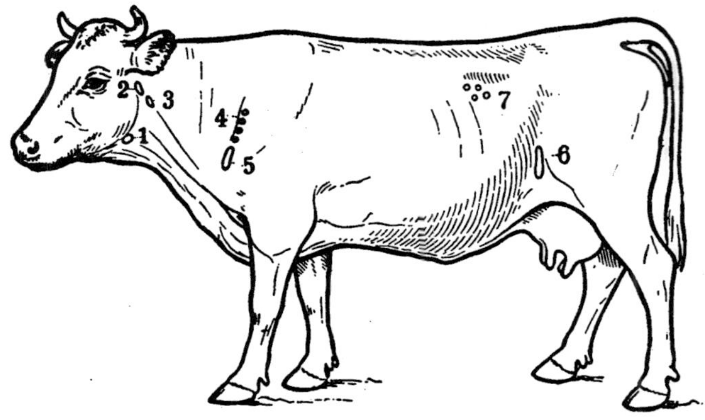

Lymph glands of the ox accessible by external palpation.

5. The lymphatics of the shoulder (prescapular glands) are covered by the mastoido-humeralis muscle in front of the scapulo-humeral articulation.

6. The precrural glands lie at the anterior border of the tensor fascia lata muscle; distinctly visible in cattle.

7. In the upper part of the flank of the ox four or five follicles as large as a lentil can frequently be felt subcutaneously.

8. The deep inguinal glands lie in the crural canal covering the crural vessels.

[The superficial inguinal glands in the male animal at the neck of the scrotum on each side of the penis in the sheath. In the female as follows:]

9. The retromammary glands (glands of the udder) are especially well developed in the cow and are situated, behind and above the udder.

10. The mesenteric, lumbar and sacral glands of the horse and cow can be examined per rectum. In the former the bowel should be evacuated by means of a cathartic; for the latter it is at least advisable to do so.

In the healthy horse we can distinctly feel the intermaxillary glands, in the healthy ox the precrural glands, and no others; if any of the other glands are distinctly palpable we assume that they are enlarged.

The intermaxillary lymphatic glands of the horse are sometimes extirpated in order to subject them to a special macroscopical, or microscopical and bacteriological examination. For diagnostic purposes we resort to it in glanders only. We operate on the standing animal and anesthetize according to Schleich's method.

15. The Blood.

The examination of the blood is of importance in a few rare cases only. A microscopical examination to determine

Fig. 54.

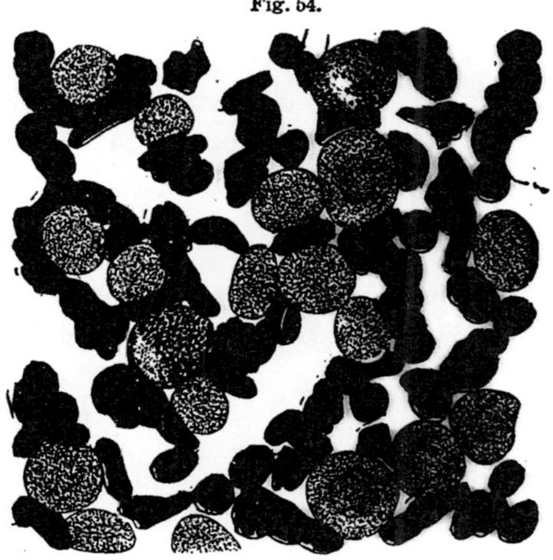

Leucemic Blood.

the presence of certain infectious diseases is of value only in anthrax and Rothlauf in pigs, and even in these diseases the circulating blood contains only few organisms. However, in Texas fever it is of diagnostic importance, and in constitutional blood diseases it is equally invaluable.

The best way to obtain the necessary blood is to make a slight incision into the lip, with the point of a knife, observing care not to stretch the skin during the operation. If a larger quantity of blood is desired a hypodermic needle, inserted into the jugular vein, answers the purpose better. [As far as annoyance of the animal is concerned, tapping the jugular vein is preferable in all cases.] In practice we may limit ourselves to the microscopical examination; for this purpose a single drop of blood, placed directly on the glass slip or cover, will serve the purpose. From this drop we can make a few cover glass preparations, allow them to dry, take them home, fix, stain and examine them at leisure; or we may add a 0.3% solution of sodium chloride and examine the blood in its fluid condition. Exact blood examinations are difficult and must be carried out with such care and minuteness that the practitioner is obliged to get along with the results of the simplest methods. For those who care to take up the study of blood examinations in detail we recommend "Jacksch-Klinische Diagnostik."

Fig. 55.

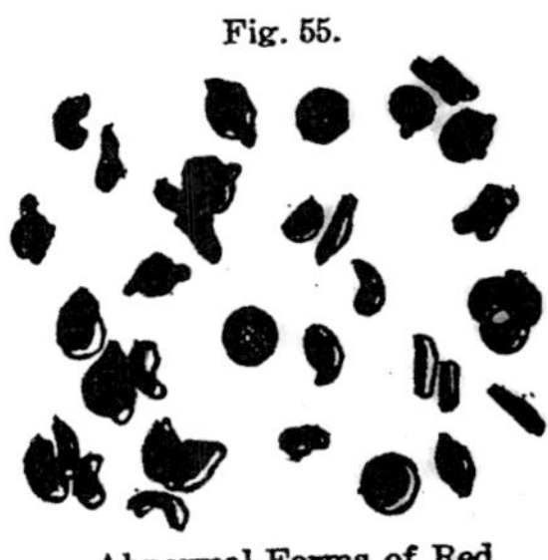

Abnormal Forms of Red Corpuscles.

Number of blood corpuscles. The absolute number of blood corpuscles in a given amount of blood can only be determined with the aid of special blood-counting apparatus (Thoma-Zeiss). According to the investigations of Storch, the number and proportion of red and white corpuscles per cubic millimeter are as follows:

	Red Corpuscles.	White Corpuscles.	Proportion.
Stallions	8.2 millions	10,500	1:780
Geldings	7.6 "	11,000	1:690
Mares	7.1 "	9,900	1:720
Colts	9.3 "	14,000	1:670
Bulls	6.5 "	7,800	1:820
Steers	6.7 "	9,400	1:720
Cows	5.5 "	8,200	1:660
Calves	8.5 "	15,700	1:550
Dogs	5.4 "	3,100-2,800	——

Since the results of these investigations show that considerable variations occur under normal conditions, extreme variations alone can be regarded as being of importance.

An increase in the number of red corpuscles has been observed in serious general diseases with fatal termination: pulmonary gangrene, angina, pleuro-pneumonia.

A decrease in the number of erythrocytes occurs in essential anemia, hydremia, leukemia, and particularly in pernicious anemia.

Shape of the red blood corpuscles. We usually group them as follows:

1. Normal red corpuscles, without nucleus.
2. Nucleated erythrocytes.
    a. Normoblasts of normal size.
    b. Megaloblasts, two or three times the size of normal red corpuscles.
    c. Gigantoblasts, still larger than the megaloblasts.
    d. Microblasts, smaller than the normoblasts.

When the normal blood corpuscles deviate from their usual biconcave form they are called poikilocytes. Similarly altered nucleated red corpuscles are called poikiloblasts.

The red corpuscles frequently undergo considerable change in form in the course of preparation for microscopic examination. This must always be borne in mind when differentiating between the different groups.

Varieties of the white corpuscles. According to Ehrlich and his pupils the white corpuscles are classified as follows:

1. Lymphocytes. These are from 6 to 9 micra in diameter, with a single, large, well-defined nucleus containing an abundance of chromatin. They stain with basic aniline dyes, the protoplasm absorbing more of the stain than the nucleus.

2. Large Mononuclear Leucocytes. These are 12 to 15 micra in diameter, contain a large, not well-defined single nucleus with little chromatin, and homogeneous, basophile protoplasm.

Transition forms occupy a position between the large mononuclear leucocytes and the polynuclear leucocytes, their nucleus being divided into two or three sections. They resemble the mononuclears in their affinity for stains.

3. Polynuclear Leucocytes. These are 10 to 12 micra in diameter, are provided with a slender but broken and irregular nucleus containing an abundance of chromatin and a finely granular, opaque, neutrophile protoplasm.

4. Eosinophile Leucocytes. These are 12 to 15 micra in diameter, the body of the cell is filled with large roundish granules which have an exceptional affinity for eosin and other acid stains. They have one or two nuclei which are packed in between the granules. The nuclei contain an abundance of chromatin.

5. Mast Cells. These vary in size up to that of the eosinophyles, they have clumsy nuclei of various forms containing little chromatin, and basophyle, coarsely granular protoplasm.

According to Wiendick the varieties of leucocytes occur in the following proportions in the blood of the horse:

	Percentage.	Actual No. per cubic centimeter.
1. Lymphocytes	35-45	2500-3500
2. Mononuclear Leucocytes	1.5-3.5	150-300
3. Neutrophyle Polynuclear Leucocytes	50-70	4000-5000
4. Acidophyle Leucocytes	1.5-5.0	200-350
5. Mast Cells (Basophyle leucocytes)	0.2-0.7	20-60

It is not unusual to observe even greater variations than those shown in the table.

A temporary increase in the actual number of leucocytes (hyperleucocytosis) may occur after feeding and in animals in advanced pregnancy. Such an increase is also observed in the course of all infectious inflammatory processes, especially during the formation of abscesses in the course of strangles.

The actual number of leucocytes is reduced (hypoleucocytosis) permanently in the course of pernicious anemia. In this disease the relative proportion of red corpuscles is less than normal.

The normal color of blood serum is a light golden yellow (straw color). After the destruction or breaking down of a large number of red corpuscles their coloring matter is dissolved in the plasma of the blood and is partially converted into methemoglobin. This causes a reddening of the serum (Hemoglobinemia). The presence of the coloring matter of the muscles may produce a similar result.

Diseases of the Blood.

Essential (idiopathic) anemia. Bloodlessness. Consists in a diminishment of the quantity of blood without a determinable cause. Blood pale and coagulates poorly. Mucous membranes pale and low temperature. Pulse small, heart tones metallic sound. Appetite poor. Tendency to dropsical swellings. General weakness. Mostly in young animals.

Leucemia. Chronic alterations of the blood and increase in number of white corpuscles. Animals are languid, lazy, sweat easily, pale mucous membranes. Appetite grows less, pulse increases, small. Heart tones, metallic sound. Enlargement of lymphatic glands usually present. Sometimes ecchymotic hemorrhages in the mucous membranes.

Infectious anemia of the horse. Transmissible, usually fatal disease, course acute or chronic. Fever, 40.5° C. [104.9° F.] appears after a period of incubation of 5-9 days, subsiding as the disease advances. Marked weakness, especially in hind quarters, dirty yellowish red conjunctiva, some petecheae. Impaired appetite, emaciation, swellings. Red corpuscles reduced in numbers.

Hemoglobinuria of cattle. An acute non-contagious infectious disease of cattle caused by the presence of the protozoon Pyroplasma bigeminum in the blood, and characterized by hemoglobinuria. About 12 days after the animals have been on an infected pasture, the first symptoms appear—fever, loss of appetite, diarrhea. Urine light to dark red, very foamy, urination painful. Urine contains hemoglobin and coagulates into a gelatinous mass when boiled. Gait stiff and clumsy, often attended with pain. Also anemia, icterus, general debility, continuous lying down, edematous swelling of head and neck.

The cause of the disease is found in the blood in the form of a protozoon called Pyroplasma bigeminum. The latter has a roundish form which may become very irregular as a result of ameboid movement.

When fully developed they are found in the red corpuscles in the form of two pear shaped bodies with the narrow ends approaching each other, or in actual contact. They are 2.5-4 micra long and 1.5 to 2 micra wide. Two per cent. of the red corpuscles in the circulating blood are infected, while 50% of the red corpuscles of the capillaries of the organs contain the parasites.

The presence of the parasites is easily demonstrated by fixing smear preparations in absolute alcohol and staining with alkaline methylene blue.

Texas Fever. Is an infectious disease of cattle caused by Pyrosoma bigeminum [indirectly by the presence of Texas fever ticks, Boophilus bovis]. Period of incubation 10-15 days. High and continuous fever, rapidly progressing anemia, red corpuscles reduced in number from six million to one million per cc. Hemaglobinuria. Fatal termination the rule.

P y r o s o m a b i g e m i n u m is a minute pale protozoon of a roundish form found in the red corpuscles. It possesses ameboid movement and can therefore assume irregular shapes. When fully developed the parasites occur as two pear-shaped bodies with

Fig. 56.

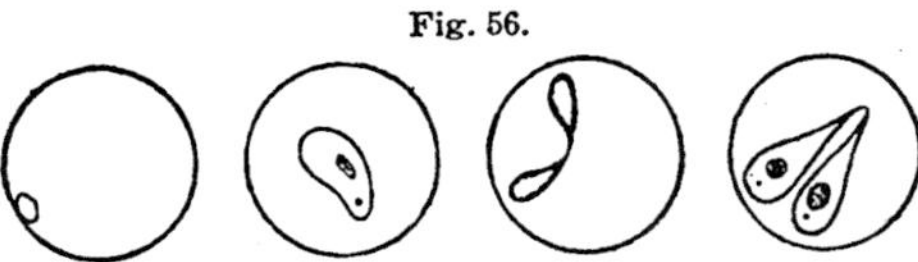

Different stages of development of Pyrosoma bigeminum in red blood corpuscles.

their pointed ends, converging. They are 2.5 to 4 micra long and 1.5 to 2 micra wide. In the circulating blood 1 to 2% of the blood corpuscles are infected, in the capillaries of the various organs more than half of them contain the parasites.

Malaria A non-contagious infectious disease caused by Plasmodium malariae. Remittent fever, pronounced icterus, petechiae, cerebral depression, small rapid pulse. Loss of appetite, increased thirst, dark-colored urine staining white hair yellow. The malaria parasites which occur in the blood constitute a special group of protozoons. They differ from the Pyrosoma in being pigmented. They may be stained with methylene blue. They are bright roundish bodies with distinct outline, occurring singly in the red blood corpuscles.

Flagellosis of horses. Mal de Caderas. Gradually rising recurrent fever rarely exceeding 40° C. (104° F.) Rapid emaciation in spite of good appetite. Paralysis of the hind quarters, bladder and rectum. Edema, hemoglobinuria, continuous lying down, coma, death. The specific cause of the disease, Trypanosoma equina (Flagellata) is found in the blood as an actively motile parasite. Smear preparations may be stained in 15-20 minutes with carbol-fuchsin to which has been added one-third volume of glycerine. Magenta red, however, is a better stain. The parasite has the form of a whip lash and is three or four times the length

[Malkmus regards this disease and hemoglobinuria of cattle (Europe) as very probably identical.]—Translators.

of the diameter of a red blood corpuscle. The convex border of the body contains a delicate membrane which extends to the end of the body, forming a tail. The body of the parasite contains bright round granules which do not take the stain. Very destructive in South America.

Fig. 57.

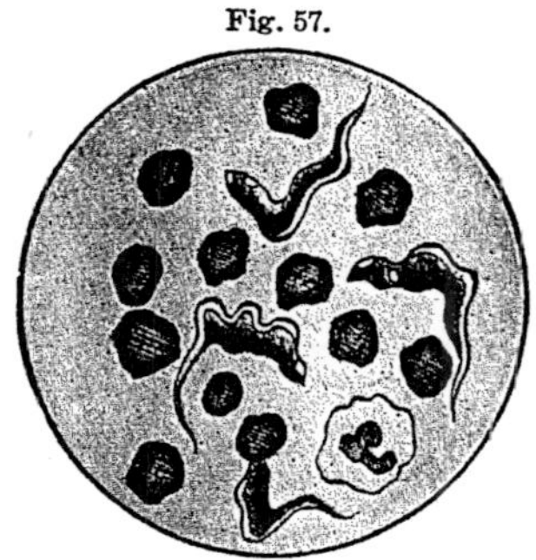

Nagana, Tsetse Disease, Surra. Occurs in cattle, solidungula, camels, dogs and cats. This is a pernicious anemia caused by Trypanosoma Evansi (introduced into the tissues through the medium of the tsetse fly). Fever, muscular weakness, edema, affection of the eyes, pronounced anemia. A flaggellate parasite, like the above, 20 to 40 micra long, 1 to 2.5 micra in diameter, actively motile.

Dourine. Maladie de coit. Lesions of the genital organs and skin.

Trypanosoma equiperdum in the blood.

INDEX.

Abdomen 140, 153.
Abnormal sensitiveness 156.
Accumulation of food 153, 161.
Achorion Schoenleinii, see Favus 55.
Acne contagiosa equor, see Canadian horsepox 57.
Actinomycoma 149.
Actinomycosis 143.
Albuminuria 67, 184, 185.
Albumosuria 186.
Alkalies, craving for 141.
Alopecia 45, **51.**
Alveolar periostitis 144.
Anemia 47, 60, **249.**
Anesthesia 213.
Anamnesis 18.
Anasarca 46.
Angina pharyngea **171.**
Ante-and post-partum paresis 38.
Anthrax **72,** 240.
Anus 105.
Apoplexy 216, **219.**
Appetite 141.
Arteries 81.
Ascites 40.
Ascarides 63.
Atelectasis 27, 130.
Attitude 33.
Auscultation 29.
—of abdomen 161.
—of heart 86.
—of lungs 130.
Azoturia 37, 42.
Bacillus pyelonephritis 199.
Balkiness 229.
Bird lice 52.
Blackleg **58.**
Bladder, diseases of 176.
—, examination of 200.
Blind staggers **219,** 221.
Blood 245, 246.
Blood sweating, **51.**
Blowing sound 100, 106.
Bodily temperature 63.
Bovine pest **58.**
Broken back 37.
Bronchial catarrh **136.**
Bronchiectases 129.
Bronchitis 107, **137.**
—verminosa **137.**
Bruits, anemic 90.
—, diastolic 87.
—, inorganic 88.
—, systolic, 87.

Cachexia 39.
Canadian horsepox **57.**
Carbonate of lime 193.
Cardiac dullness 85.
Catarrh of maxillary sinuses **136.**
—, of gutteral pouches 136.
Caverns in lungs 129.
Cerebral congestion **218.**
—depression 210.
—hemorrhage **219.**
Cerebrospinal meningitis 38, 42, **220.**
Chills 67.
Choleurea 189.

Circulatory apparatus 75.
Coital exanthema 208.
Colic 42, 164, **172.**
Collapse, temperature of 71.
Colostral milk 205.
Colpitis 207.
Coma 211.
Condition 39.
Conformation 40.
Congestion, cerebral **218.**
Conjunctiva 59.
Constipation 162, 164, 174.
Convulsions 213.
Cough 117.
—, return impulse of 120.
Cracked pot resonance 129.
Cramp of the neck 38, 42, 214.
Crisis 71.
Crusts 51.
Cystitis **201.**

Defecation 163, 164, 218.
Degultition, difficulties of 145.
Diabetes 180.
—insipidus **202.**
—mellitus **202.**
Diaphragm, rupture of 129.
Diarrhea 155, 164.
Dicrotic pulse 81.
Differential diagnosis 16.
Digestive apparatus 140.
Dilatation of the heart **91.**
Direct diagnosis 16.
Dislocation of bowel **129,** 173.
Distemper of dogs 140, 213, **216.**
—of horses 139.
Distoma, eggs of 169.
Diverticula of esophagus 150, **173.**
Dizziness 212, **219.**
Drowsiness 211.
Dropsy 46.
Dummies 31, 34, 219, 221.
Dyspepsia **172.**
Dyspnea 34, 102.
Dysuria 178.

Ecchymoses 113, 114, 147.
Echinococcus disease **137.**
Eclampsia **219.**
Eczema **51.**
Edema 23, 47, 58.
—of glottis 136.
—collateral 47.
Emphysema 24, 48.
—, alveolar **131.**
—, cutaneous 24, 48.
—, interstitial **137.**
—, of skin 47.
—, septic 48.
Encephalitis 34.
Endocarditis, acute and chronic **91.**
Endometritis **207.**
Enteritis, hemorrhagic 167.
Enteroliths 159.
Epilepsy 214, **219**, 228, 229.
Epistaxis 135.
Epithelial casts 199.
—cells 198.
Eructation 151.
Esbach's albuminimeter 185.
Esophagus 149.
Excitability, abnormal 222.
Exhalations 105.
Expired air, odor of **106.**

Facies hypocratica 42.
Facial nerve, paralysis of 216.
Fagopyrism **51.**
Fainting 212.
Favus **55.**

Feces 163, 165.
—, retention of 164.
—, voiding of 164.
—, volume of 165.
Fermentation test 192.
Fever 66, 68.
—, catarrhal 139.
Fowl cholera 73.
—, diphtheria 140.
—, pest 73.
—curve 68.
—, types of 70.
Fluctuation 24.
Flagellosis 250.
Fleas 52.
Food, manner of taking 142.
Foot and mouth disease **56.**
Foot eczema **51.**
Foreign bodies in intestines 174.
—in esophagus **171.**
Fowl cholera **73.**
Friction bruits of pleura 135.

Garglings 101.
Garget 207.
Gastro-enteritis **172.**
Gastro-intestinal catarrh. **172.**
Glanders 139.
—ulcer 114.
—cicatrices 114.
Gmelin's test 190.
Gram's method **199.**
Granular casts 199.
Granule casts 198.
Grape sugar 192.
Groaning 101.
Grunting 101.
Guttie of ox 34, **173.**

Habitus 32.
Hematopinus **52.**
Hair coat 44.
—, shedding of **45.**
Heart 83.
—beat 84.
—sounds 86, **87.**
Heave line 104.
Heaves 224.
Hematuria 188, **201.**
Hemidrosis 46, 51.
Hemiplegia 104.
Hemiplegia, laryngis sinistra 136.
Hemoglobinuria 187, 188. 201, **249.**
Hepatization 27, 129.
Herpes tonsurans 55.
Hippuric acid 195.
Hives 51.
Hog cholera 72.
Hyaline casts 198.
Hydrocephalus 214, **218.**
Hypesthesia 213.
Hyperemia of kidneys, passive **201.**
Hyperesthesia 213.
Hypertrophy of heart **91.**
Hyperidrosis 46.
Hyperthermia 219.
Hypidrosis 46.

Icterus 61, 62, 212.
Immobility 221.
Impaction of intestines 158.
—, rectum 216.
Incarceration 158.
Incontinentia urinae **201.**
Indican 188.
Influenza **72.**
Inoculation 230, 234.
—for anthrax, etc., 240.
—for glanders 235.
—for rabies 241.
—for tuberculosis 231.
Insufficiency 88.
—of mitral valves 91.
—of semi-lunar valves 88, 91.
—of tricuspid valves 91.
Intermaxillary lymph glands 115.
Intestinal catarrh 172.
—evacuations 163.
—gases 170.
—noises or sounds **161.**
—peristalsis 163.
Intoxication 19.
Invagination 35, 159.
Ischury 179.

Kidneys, passive hyperemia of **201.**
Kyphosis 43.

Laryngeal catarrh 136.
Laryngeal fremitus 123.
Laryngitis, croupous **136.**
Laryngoscopy 122.
Leucocytosis 248.
Leucemia **249.**
Lice 52.
Licking disease 173.
Lime casts 170.
Liver 170.
Lockjaw **220,** see tetanus
Loco weed poisoning 176.
Lordosis 43.
Louse flies 52.
Lumbago 37, **42,** see azoturia.
Lungs, congestion of 137.
—, gangrene of 137.
—, edema of 137.
Lupinosis **175.**
Lymphatic glands 243.
Lysis 71.

Mast cells 248.
Macula 50.
Mal de Cederas 250.
Mal du coit **208.**
Malaria 250.
Malignant catarrhal fever **139.**
—carbuncle 47.
—edema **58.**
Malingerers 36.
Mallein inoculation 235.
Malleus 139.
Mange **54.**
—, acarus **55.**
—, psoroptic **54.**
—, sarcoptic **54.**
—, sacoptic, of fowls **54**
—, symbiotic **54.**
Mastication 141.
Mastitis **207.**
Melanosarcoma 149.
Microcytes 248.
Milk fever see parturient paresis 38.
Mites 52.
Mold poisoning, see mycosis, 147.

Monoplegia 216.
Morbus maculosus, see purpura hemorrhagica.
Motility 210, 213.
Mouth cavity 146.
Mouth speculum **148.**
Mycosis 147.
Mydriasis 217.
Mucous click 100.
Muscular rheumatism **42.**
Muscular sense 215.
Myocarditis, acute **91.**

Nagana 251.
Nasal catarrh **135.**
—discharge 93.
—mucous membrane 113.
—tone, see mucous click 100.
Nephritis 201.
Nettle rash 57.
Nervous system 218.
Nodules, see papules 50, 114.
Nymphomania 202.

Obesity 39.
Ocular vertigo 212.
Estrus ovis, larva of 109.
Opisthotonus 213.
Orthotonus 213.
Osteomalacea 43.
Overfeeding 153, 156.
Oxalate of lime 195.

Palpation 23.
—of bowels per rectum 156.
Panting 99.
Papules 50.
Paraplegia 104, 216.
Paralysis 215.
—of bladder 179.
—of facial nerve **219.**
—of the larynx 136.
—of esophagus and pharynx 145, 171.
—of paunch 150.
—of recurrent nerve **226.**
Parasites, intestinal 169.
—in cavities of head 135.
Paresis 215.
Parturient paresis 38, **71, 220.**
Pathognomic symptoms **14.**
Paunch, paresis of 156.
—, peristalsis of 156.
—, gases in 153.
Pentastonum tenioides **109.**
Percussion 24.
Percussion, field of **126.**
—of abdomen 159.
Pericarditis 85, **92.**
—, traumatic, of ox **92.**
Peritoneal hernia 159.
Peritonitis 34, 174.
Pernicious anemia **246.**
Peruphigus acuta 57.
Petechia 113, 114, 147.
Pharyngitis 149, **171.**
Pleuritis 34, 85, **138.**
Pleurodynia 34, 137.
Pleuropneumonia of cattle **139.**
—of the horse 138.
Pneumonia 128.
—, catarrhal **137.**
Pneumothorax **131.**
Poikilocytes **247.**
Polyarthritis **42.**
Priapism 202.
Proctitis 147.
Prurigo 219, **51.**
Pseudo fluctuation **24.**
Psychic functions **210.**

Ptyalism **171.**
Pulmonary, congestion and edema **137.**
—hemorrhage 137.
—gangrene **137.**
—resonance 128.
Pulse 67, 73, 75.
Pumping of flanks 104.
Purpura hemorrhagica 57, **114.**
Pustules 50.
Pyemia **71.**
Pyelonephritis **201.**
Pyrosoma bigeminum 250.
Pyrocatechin in horse urine 192.

Quality of percussion sounds 27.
Quibbing 144.

Rabies **216,** 220.
Rachitis 43.
Rales 133.
—, crepitant 134.
—, dry 134.
—, moist 134.
Reflex excitability 217.
Reflex spasms 214.
Regions of the body 21.
Regurgitation 127, 131.
Resistance in percussion 28
Respiration, types of 99.
—, amphoric 133.
—, bronchial 133.
—, vague or indefinite 133.
—, vesicular 131.
—, Gheyne-Stokes 98.
Respiratory apparatus 93.
Retentio urinae **201.**
Return sound 120.
Riding school movements 214.
Rinderpest **174.**
Rinderseuche 240.
Ringworm **55.**
Risus sardonicus 214.
Roaring 98, 136, **226.**
Rothlauf 212, 245.
Rumination 150.

Saliva, secretion of **147.**
Satyriasis 202.
Saw-horse attitude 34, **214.**
Scabs 51.
Scalma **138.**
Sensibility 210, 212.
Septicemia 71, **73.**
Serum diagnosis 237, 238.
Sexual apparatus **202.**
—desire 202.
Sheep pox **57.**
—, braxy 73.
Signalment **31.**
Skin 43.
—, color of 49.
—, moisture of 45.
—, odors of 50.
—, reflexes of 217.
—, sclerosis of 50.
Skoliosis 43.
Sleepiness 211.
Sneezing 100.
Snoring 100.
Snorting 99.
Somnolency **211.**
Sopor 211.
Spasms 213.
Spinal paralysis 37, **216.**
Spinal meningitis 214.
—, reflexes 217.
Spine, fracture of 37, **216.**

Spleen **171.**
Stasis 46.
Starvation 154.
Stenosis of air passages 226.
—of cardiac valves 88, 89.
—of esophagus **171.**
Stenotic laryngeal tone 101.
Stethoscope 29.
Stomacace 147
Stomatitis **171.**
—pustulosa contagiosa **175.**
Strangles **139,** see distemper.
Stranguria 178.
Strongylus filaria 137.
Submaxillary lymph glands 93, 115.
Suffusions 113.
Sulphate of lime 196.
Summer surfeit **51.**
Surra 251.
Sweating 45, 46.
Sweeny 48.
Swine erysipelas 73.
Swine plague **65, 72.**
Symptoms 12.
Syncope 212.

Teeth 148.
—, caries of 106.
—, diseases of **172.**
—, gnashing of the 144.
Temperament 40.
Tetanus 37, 219.
Texas fever 73, 245, 250.
Thirst, see "Desire for water" p. 142.
Ticks 52.
Torsion of colon 159.
Torsio uteri **207.**
Trembling 213.
Trichodectes 52.
Trichoerhexis nodosa 56.
Tricophyton tonsurans 55.
Triple phosphate 196.
Trismus 213.
Trommer's test 192.
Tubercle bacilli 111.
Tuberculin test 231.
Tuberculosis 138, 203, 207.
—, of brain 220.
Tumors in cavities of head **136.**
Turnsick 212, 214, 219.
Tympanitis 173.
—acuta, **151,** 173.
—chronica **151,** 173.
Tzetse disease 251.

Udder 204, 206
Ulcers 147.
—catarrhal or erosion 114.
Upper air passages 112.
Uremia 212.
Urethral calculi 200.
Uric acid 195.
Urinary apparatus 176.
—casts 198.
Urination 176.
Urine, sediment in 194.
—, odor of 182.
Urolithiasis 202.
—, voiding of 177.
Urticaria **57.**

Vaginal mucous membrane 204.
Vaginitis **207.**
Valvular diseases **91.**
Veins 81.
—, undulation of jugular 82.
Venous pulse 83.
Verminous bronchitis 137.

Vertigo 212, 228, 229.
Vesicles 50.
Vesicular eruption 203, 208.
Vesicular murmur 131.
—respiration 132.
Voice, change in 121.
Vomiting 151.
—in horses 151.

Water, desire for 142.
Whistling 102, 227.
Woody tongue 143.
Wool eating 169.
Wool in feces 169.
Wheezing 100.
Wild-und Rinder-seuche 58, 240.

Yawn 100.